ONE ANIMAL AMONG MANY

GAIA, GOATS & GARLIC

DAVID WALTNER-TOEWS, DVM, PhD

NC Press Limited

Toronto 1991

Cover Design by Jerry Ginsberg
Front Cover Photo:
    ©1991 The Shepherds Project, by permission,
    Ontario Veterinary College
Rear Cover Photo: ©1990 Tim Sullivan

Canadian Cataloguing in Publication Data

Waltner-Toews, David, 1948-
One Animal Among Many

ISBN 1-55021-067-X

1. Livestock - Ecology. 2. Agricultural Ecology. 3. Human Ecology
I. Title.

S589.7.W35 1992   630'.2'745   C91-095777-0

We would like to thank the Ontario Arts Council and the Canada
Council for their assistance in the production of this book.
New Canada Publications, a division of NC Press Limited,
Box 452, Station A, Toronto, Ontario, Canada, M5W 1H8.

Printed and bound in Canada

Contents

ACKNOWLEDGEMENTS

One Animal Among Many and *Old Animal: New Thoughts,* were originally part of one piece, *One Animal Among Many: Veterinarians in the Global Community,* first presented as the D.L.T Smith Lecture at the University of Saskatchewan in 1988 and later published in the *Canadian Veterinary Journal.*

Potbellied Pigs and the Natural Order, is reprinted courtesy of *Harrowsmith Country Life* magazine, Ferry Road, Charlotte, Vermont, U.S.A. 05445.

Ecological Agriculture was presented to the Ontario Ministry of Agriculture and Food, Animal Industry Branch (1991).

What's a Small Abattoir Good For? was a presentation made to the OMAF Livestock Inspection Branch (1991).

Little Bo-Peep Meets David Suzuki was a presentation made to the Ontario Sheep Marketing Agency (1991).

Creation and Extinction: A Meditation was a presentation made to the Rockway Mennonite Church.

The following have never been published or presented: *Animal Rights: Gaia Rights; Thrush: The Case of the Singing Feet.*

The remainder were published in, and appear by courtesy of *Harrowsmith Magazine,* 7 Queen Victoria Road, Camden East, Ontario K0K 1J0.

All Essays have been revised for this book, some of them substantially, and many of the titles have been changed.

This collection of essays is dedicated to Mary Oyer and Mary Ellen Bender, who taught me that music, philosophy, literature, science and medicine were all of a piece, and that what lives as a whole we sunder at our intellectual and biological peril.

PREFACE: OVER THE FENCE

A fence, for a rural veterinarian, is a wonderful device. It serves at once as a podium from which to preach the virtues of good animal husbandry, a lectern from which to scold the wayward farmer, a barrier over which one can flee from a raging cow, a wall at which to lament the death of a duck or a pony, and an excuse for conversation. "Well, guess we might as well pause here," one might say, arriving at a wooden fence. From there, one can lead a client's eyes away from some assuredly paltry medical failure, and out to the wonder of crops ripening, cows at pasture, and beyond, perhaps to a sunrise.

There are moments when the direct, no-nonsense approach is called for, when the modern biomedical way of looking at things comes into its own, in cranking a stubborn calf through a tight birth canal, or in the midst of castrating a two-year-old Belgian horse. There are people who delight in the pontifications which may spring off the wall at such moments: this animal has penicillin deficiency, or, your bill is $257.63. I too have been trained in these matters, but that is not the matter of these essays.

Such veterinary advice as may appear from time to time in these ruminations is strictly over the fence. If you take my advice, and it doesn't work, and then you come grinding your teeth back to me, be assured that I will say that I may have been wrong. Like as not, I shall refer to Solomon, who said:
> There are three things which are too wonderful for me,
> Four which I do not understand:
> The way of an eagle in the sky,
> The way of a serpent on a rock,
> The way of a ship in the middle of the sea,
> And the way of a man with a maid.

And then I shall lean over the fence and point out to you how the alfalfa is flowering, and how the cattle love it in the succulence of its youth, but how they disdain it in its stiff and bitter old age. I will tell you how they can inflate with gas to the point of death from their indulgence in youthful alfalfa, and what this might mean in terms of politics or social values. And by the time I have finished you will, I hope, have forgotten why it was that you came to me in the first place, and perhaps you will even be willing to pay me for my professional advice, and we shall both go our ways feeling a little better about life.

David Waltner-Toews, DVM, PhD

Guelph, Ontario, Canada

PART I:

GAIA

ONE ANIMAL AMONG MANY

According to some commentators on the Jewish Talmud, God tried creation twenty-six times before this one. All of the early attempts failed. "Let's hope it works this time," said the Creator, sending us on our strange, beautiful -- and uncertain -- journey. It is a hope many of us mutter to ourselves quite often these days. But hope without action is only a cynical parody of hope; real hope carries with it the responsibility to bring that hope to fruition. Real hope is thus self-fulfilling, a positive feedback loop. But real despair, which grips us too easily these days, is also self-fulfilling, and carries with it its own downward spiral. The greatest challenge of our time is to make the leap of imagination -- for that, ultimately is what it must be -- from the down-slide to the upward climb.

To the extent that humans are natural beings, and I would argue that we are completely so, human ideas and feelings are as much natural products as the gases over swamps and the apples in the tree in my back yard. There is no way to separate into different categories human ideas about Nature and Nature's thoughts about herself. Just as we, each of us, know ourselves best insofar as we can integrate our intellectual and experiential ways of understanding, so we, collectively, can only know Nature insofar as we celebrate the mystery of our global inter-connectedness.

We live in one world, in which there are many ways of knowing. Scientists who study the evolution of the earth have spent a great deal of energy in recent decades exploring the waves of extinction and evolutionary flowering which have preceded our present age. Evolutionary biologists and ecologists tell us (but act as if they do not believe it) that we are one with nature.

These are things that some people -- mystics and prophets -- have celebrated for centuries. One does not need to resort to unbelievable phenomena to explain this. We are, after all, the product of that evolution and this ecological web, and thus, in a very real sense, incorporate those waves of destruction and creation in the very structure of our body cells and organs. At the level of mechanism, mysticism is built into the biological and social DNA of our beings, and is as natural and as understandable (!) as a cat's behaviour. It would indeed be surprising if we, collectively, did not intuitively understand everything that scientists now so clearly and explicitly elucidate long before science was "invented". In this very real sense, everything in the world is "natural" -- industrial polluters and Greenpeace alike -- for there is nothing outside of Nature.

The excessive multiplication of humans beyond the ability of the environment to sustain us, and the excessive plundering of the world's energy sources, particularly for military purposes, are finally bringing the reality of our interconnectedness home. I hope it's not to late for what is after all only common sense to prevail. Neither science nor religion have served us particularly well in this regard. The Darwinian principle that the fittest are those that reproduce the best is a simple re-statement of the Biblical directive to be fruitful and multiply (or perhaps the Biblical directive was a religious statement of a principle our evolutionary forbears saw clearly millennia before Darwin). Whatever the source of our belief in the virtues of copulatory multiplication, we should by now realize that we have ably fulfilled our evolutionary/ religious mandate, that just because a little bit of being fruitful is good doesn't mean that lots of fruitfulness is better, and that we can now move on to commandment number next, that is, to love our suffering neighbours enough to promote the greening of the planet.

Science has given -- is giving -- us a wonderfully detailed description of the structure of our world and our universe. The tragedy of our success at scientific discovery has been the arrogance that has accompanied it, the foolishness of the three blind men and the elephant. Just like the religious arrogance of the Biblical literalists and Muslim fundamentalists, it is an arrogance born of fear. Fear that we might be part of something we can never completely fathom, fear that the understanding of mechanism is not identical with the understanding of purpose, that the sum of the reductionist experts does not translate into wisdom.

Wisdom is greater than the sum of all knowledge, life is greater than the sum of her DNA, and the world is greater than the sum of her artificially designated Latin names. As we move up through various layers of earth's ecosystem, from inanimate matter to complex living beings, we find that the whole in one level (atom, molecule, cell, animal, herd, nation) is greater than the simple sum of its parts. Neither do the rules change at the global level: we, the world, Gaia, are greater than the sum of our parts.

In ancient days, we lived brutally, simply, surrounded by mystery. As modern humans we have deluded ourselves into believing that there really is a dotted line at the equator, and that a detailed description of the laws of nature explains the mystery of why those laws are so constituted. In the vision of William Blake, we have moved from innocence to experience. Few would argue that this has been, overall, a negative development. But now, after all, it is time to grow up into the "higher innocence", to see things whole again, and to lay aside the silly, infantile notions that science, religion, and politics can ultimately be explained by reference to different realities. This is not a reversion to the "old" mysticism, to religious dogmatism and deference to papal or Nobel authorities. This is calling for a new synthesis of knowledge, our greatest act of imagination, a vision of reality greater than the sum of all our individual historically and genetically conditioned thoughts.

There is one reality, one wonderful animal which is all of us together. The sooner we come to terms with that, practically, in all walks of life, the greater will be our chances of surviving to remain a recognizable part of this reality.

OLD ANIMAL: NEW THOUGHTS

We live, it seems, in a broken world. We reached toward the wonders of the world around us as a child might reach up to her grandmother's precious and delicate china cups, displayed so temptingly up there on the narrow wooden shelves. Just when we thought we could touch the deepest mysteries of life and the universe, that we had them here in our pudgy little scientific hands in all their power and beauty, they have come crashing down around us, shards and fragments everywhere. We never intended this.

We never really planned to have enough nuclear weapons to kill every person twelve times over. It was never our intention to lose six tons of topsoil for every ton of grain produced in North America, nor to shoot down civilian airliners to protect our oil supplies or some nineteenth century ideology, nor to pillage African raw materials for our own economic benefit and leave millions of children to die in our murderous wake, nor to poison our milk and vegetables and meat and chocolates and children with PBBs or DDT or radionuclides, nor to turn productive ecosystems into deserts, or drive thousands of plant and animal species into extinction, nor to drive tens of millions of people from their homes with our utopian political solutions -- capitalist and communist alike -- and our single-minded, simplistic agricultural practices. No, these were not what tempted us to reach up to that china cabinet.

We wanted beauty, and peace and dignity. We really did want nothing more, most of us, than a good life. Yet here we are, the pieces all around us, in Alaska and Bhopal and Afghanistan and St-Basile-le-Grand and the Love Canal and Armenia . . . as if the shifts in the earth's tectonic plates were not only geological, but social, political and ecological as well. And all the grandfathers and grandmothers in the world don't seem to be able to glue the pieces back together for us.

In the face of this, we may be tempted to throw up our hands in despair, or to jump at quick, Stalinesque solutions, bigger tractors to solve the farm labour problem, food irradiation to kill *Salmonella*, massive oil development and forest clearcutting to create jobs. It all seems too difficult and too complex to even begin the task of picking up each tiny fragment and fitting it back into its delicate whole. We suffer not only from the effects of a global energy burnout, but from a burnout of social conscience and personal energy. The planet is going to run down some day anyway. Why wait for the sun to fry us? Why not let it get blown up now?

We too -- you and I as individuals -- are going to die. Yet, more often than not, this knowledge, and the experience of the deaths of loved ones, is occasion for caring even more, not for caring less, or becoming careless about each other. Mortality does not obviate ethics; it shapes our ethics and gives it energy. Living with dignity. Dying with dignity. Doing unto others as we would wish that they do unto us. That is the vocabulary of human ethics. That also, faced with the prospect of planetary death, should be the language of a more global ethic. But how, with all the competing political and social claims being made on us, can we ever hope to accomplish what needs to be done?

In order for us to get motivated and energized to act we shall have to re-imagine ourselves and our place on this planet. Yet another moral tirade about how bad we are to cut down rainforests or slaughter whales simply will not do. The problem has been defined, thank you very much. We are ready for something else. Many of us have been preached to, and "saved", often enough to last a lifetime. The litany of our sins is boring and depressing. What we don't need is another set of ten commandments to stand in judgement over us; what we do need are beatitudes, blessings to motivate and energize us to walk on out into the kind of symbiotic, life-celebratory living that have carried this creation along over the past several billion years.

But where is there an ethic sufficiently universal and inspiring to help us deal with our fragmented sphere? The decisions we are making today seem to range far beyond the capacities of traditional western moral theories to deal with. Historically, our ethical decisions have always been framed in terms of other *people*, and have never seemed to carry the same global weight that they do today. To say that we should love and all else will fall into place may be true -- but love whom or what? family, friends, enemies, ecosystems, baby seals, our way of life, our country, our work?. . . We act morally toward those of whom we can conceive -- whether we know them in person, or through the written word, or through visual images. In order to act morally toward the earth, we need a vision of that earth as our neighbour, a living vision to excite our moral senses.

The moral strategy of much of North American society is based on the notion that we should simply "do what we do best", or "what we are trained to do", and leave the rest to other "experts". Everything then will fall into place. Zen Buddhism, Christianity -- just about any religious idea, when translated into the American idiom, falls into this trap: centre yourself and find salvation in the careful maintenance of your motorcycle (or your garden, or your soul). In any case, this strategy says, we will have done what we can. It won't be our fault if the world goes to the cockroaches. We, at least, are among the elect, the righteous. Inherently, there is nothing wrong, in fact there is everything right, about doing the best, most careful work that we can. But like horses with blinders on, we may win the race only to find that the grandstand, together with whatever cheering section might have appreciated our talents, has burned down. Or that the garden we have been tending so well belongs to Adolf Hitler. Or that the New Heaven which we expect God to have prepared for us is in fact the Old Earth which we have devastated for ourselves.

Some people have argued that, since everything is related to everything else, we need only consider humans in our ethical considerations. What's good for people will ultimately be good for the planet. If we, in our arrogance and ignorance and self-centered nationalisms and ideologies, destroy this planet, then we will have cut out from under ourselves the living branch which holds us and sustains us, tumbling ourselves ignominiously into the darkness of oblivion.

This reasoning is based on the traditional philosophy of moral humanism, a philosophy that has over the years exhibited tremendous plasticity, and emotional and rational power. In recent years, it has served as the basis for such books as Jonathan Schell's moving treatise on the true meaning of nuclear holocaust, *The Fate of the Earth*. It is also the reasoning used in advertisements by the World Wildlife Fund on Ontario television stations: help save our wildlife. It's part of your life support system. It's your life too.

While these arguments may finally be the ones that sway the politicians, they bother me by their appeal to selfishness. They may be effective arguments, but are they good ethics?

Animal rights activists, who go beyond moral humanism to a philosophy which has been called humane moralism, would have us extend humanistic concerns to other animals. If an animal is capable of suffering, it is argued, then we should not inflict suffering on that animal. I have no quarrel with that.

The animal rights philosophers like Peter Singer have certainly stimulated us and enlarged our vision. We are no longer alone, huddled around our fire in the cosmic wilderness. We at least have the comfort of our dogs and cats and horses and cows. And maybe a few wild animals that we have tamed away from their natural behaviours.

But still, that wilderness out there is something else, something apart from our being and our fears and our hopes, deserving of care and attention only because of its meaning for us, only insofar as it affects us and our domesticated animal friends. And if our moral outrage is based, not on knowing animals in their true sense, as pack animals, or predators, or hunted prey, but in looking into their eyes and projecting onto them our suffering, then how, ultimately, can we bring ourselves to care deeply about the millions of bacteria and insects that are much more essential to the earth's survival -- to our survival -- than any of us mammals?

While moral humanism and humane moralism can be used as a base to argue that we should treat the earth with care, neither of them lead us to believe that the earth and all that is in it are deserving of ethical considerations in and of themselves. We may erase the justifications for exploitation based on sex, religion, race, sexual preference and even species, but we are still, by these arguments, allowing that violence against non-sentient nature is permissible. And by this, I would argue that we still have not fully grasped the scientific discoveries of the last one hundred years, that, though we differ in function and complexity, we are all of one piece. Both from a naturalistic and a moral viewpoint inorganic atoms and organic minds are parts of a living whole, just as bones and brain and liver are part of the same animal.

Two very different attempts to extend our moral purview to include inanimate nature were undertaken in the first part of this century.

Aldo Leopold, in *The Sand County Almanac,* articulated a "land", or "environmental" ethic, based on esthetic and cultural needs, that included all the non-human elements of our planet. He speaks elegantly of humans living as respectful, nonviolent citizens in the larger community of nature. "A thing is right," he wrote, " when it tends to preserve the integrity, stability, and beauty of the biotic community. It is wrong when it tends otherwise." Leopold could see already in the 1940s that what was needed was an ethic than would lead each and every individual to feel a sense of moral responsibility for the world we live in.

More than any other person, Leopold laid the scientific ecological foundations for solving many of our twentieth century problems. The ideas he articulated have served as the basis for much of the environmental movement in North America, from the establishment of public parks to the preservation of endangered species. And yet there is something in Leopold's articulation that smacks of a bureaucratic call to civic responsibility, to being nice to each other, or the exhortations of a concerned scientist. It lacks the ringing inspiration that will lead us beyond our many creeds into global awareness.

A much more complex and passionate call to "love all of nature" was articulated by the French priest and paleontologist Teilhard de Chardin. In his book, "The Phenomenon of Man", de Chardin put forward what he called the "law of complexity and consciousness." According to this law, the evolution of life on earth is nothing less than a grand coalescence and self-organization of the primal subatomic particles of the universe into atoms, inorganic molecules, organic molecules, prokaryotic cells, eukaryotic cells, multicellular organisms, and in our time into multicellular organisms with increasingly complex nervous systems and brains.

This increase in "outer" or material complexity has been accompanied, at crucial thresholds, by measurable changes in the "inner" aspects of nature: in consciousness, the abilities to feel and think and, ultimately, reflect. In fact, the next stage in this embryogenesis will be the creation of a transhuman organism, not in a material sense, but in a conscious, thinking sense. Humanity's thoughts shall at once converge and "complexify" into one universal, infinitely complex thought, at which time we shall be like God. This is the meaning, according to de Chardin, of Christian redemption. All of earth is not only an evolving embryo, but a being whose beginning and end, whose Alpha and Omega, is centered on the person of God, and whose growing edge is the mind of humanity. This vision of the universe brings together not only the material and the spiritual, but the personal and the global, and as such, is much more satisfying, for those of us who expect our theories to explain reality, and not just the accumulated facts.

De Chardin's vision seems at once intensely religious and at the same time grandiosely anthropocentric; and while he places great emphasis on the development of "person", one can sometimes feel as if one were drowning in the tidal floods of evolution, lost in the garment folds of the cosmic Christ.

Recently, a less spiritualized, and perhaps more modest conception of our estate has been put forward by British scientist James Lovelock. His hypothesis, that the whole earth is a kind of living organism, or, as microbiologist Lynn Margulis has described it, a global autopoietic system, is a concept fully consonant with, but not bound by, evolutionary theory. On advice from novelist William Golding, Lovelock named it the Gaia Hypothesis, after the Greek goddess for Mother Earth.

The hypothesis posits that the biosphere is "a self-regulating entity with the capacity to keep our planet healthy by controlling the chemical and physical environment." While incorporating what many of us would view as common-sense ecology -- that everything is related to everything else, that Nature recycles everything, whether it be zoonotic disease agents, PCB's, nitrogen or people this hypothesis goes beyond that kind of synthesis to create a new paradigm. The earth's crust and the atmosphere do not merely support life by recycling nutrients, as in the view of classical biology. Rather, having given birth to life, their composition is itself in large measure the creation of that life. The mother and the child have become one, changing each other into something marvellously new.

The Gaia hypothesis was suggested to explain the structure of earth's atmosphere, which is far different than one would expect based on simple chemical equations. Of course we all remember the graphic pictures of the carbon, nitrogen, water and oxygen cycles from our first year biology books. There was the cloud up above, with the nitrogen joyriding down the lightning, and the cow with arrows extruding from her orifices and piling neatly up on the ground, and under the ground we have various bacteria from which the arrows circle back up to the ground surface again, perhaps into nodules on some legume, or perhaps into that amorphous entity, "the soil".

What many of us missed seeing in those cycles was the essential part that the living biosphere plays in actively maintaining and regulating those cycles, and how utterly dependent all life on this planet is on the maintenance of those cycles. The earth, since life first appeared on it, has developed, not something *like* a homeostatic system, but a real, functional, self-regulating, cybernetic homeostatic system.

The homeostatic mechanisms of Gaia regulate, among a myriad of other things, the oxygen content of the atmosphere, and the "body" temperature of the biosphere. Thus, while the energy output from the sun has increased some 30% over the last three and a half billion years, the temperature of the biosphere has never varied by more than a few degrees from its present levels. If atmospheric oxygen levels increased by a mere four percent, the world would be in a constant state of conflagration; if the oxygen levels dropped, we'd all suffocate. Those are only two small examples.

Various questions have been raised about the Gaia hypothesis by scientists. Is it falsifiable, and thus a true scientific hypothesis? I think the answer to that is yes. If we posit that the earth is an organism, and we have certain expectations and definitions of organisms, then we can see if the earth fulfils those expectations/definitions. Some ecologists would argue that the hypothesis is already falsified, since one of the properties of organisms is that they reproduce, and the earth does not reproduce itself. The question is sometimes posed as if it were rhetorical. In fact it is not. One could argue -- plausibly I think -- that the whole push for space exploration and colonization of other planets is not some grandiose scheme of humanity, but the simple biological urge of Gaia to reproduce.

If in the future other planets are colonized, then Gaia will have reproduced. If the colonists interbreed with other life forms in the universe, then one could argue that not only has a kind of yeast-like "budding" taken place, but so has sexual reproduction at the global scale. The fact that earth has not yet reproduced is to be expected since, in terms of Gaia's life expectancy, which would seem at the outside to parallel that of the sun, we are still in an embryo, and no one expects embryos to reproduce themselves. If we take a larger, universal view, we may even speak of a population of Gaias -- all the living planets everywhere in the universe; the fact that we aren't aware of them may simply reflect, on a grander scale, the biological phenomenon that the cells in one body are not aware of the cells in other bodies. An articulate discussion of these questions appears in a book by Lynn Margulis and Dorion Sagan entitled *Microcosmos: Four Billion Years of Evolution From Our Microbial Ancestors.*

The Gaia hypothesis is deeply satisfying because it can be interpreted at scientific and social and moral levels simultaneously.

It generates useful scientific and moral questions within a holistic framework which is more useful than many traditional approaches. The international "Green" movement, for instance, can be seen as a natural phenomenon of Nature, a physiological response of the Gaian body to correct the excesses of the past one hundred years. James Lovelock has argued, forcefully, that "pollution" is natural. I would argue, on the same basis, that the anti-pollution movement is an equally natural correction to that, and in fact serves as another piece of supporting evidence for the Gaia hypothesis itself.

One of the remarkable features of this global organism is how resilient it is. Early life on earth developed in a chemically reducing atmosphere, without oxygen. The buildup of oxygen in the atmosphere, which made possible life as we know it today, was, at the time it occurred, a global catastrophe resulting in mass extinctions of organisms. In terms of classical Darwinism and ecology, we would say that some organisms survived and adapted to the new environment. The Gaia hypothesis takes a larger view. Not only did some organisms "pre-adapted" to an oxidizing atmosphere survive, but Gaia herself, the global, living embryo, adapted and survived.

There have been several global catastrophes and extinctions since that time, including that of the dinosaurs, which may have been caused by earth's collision with a meteor. Whatever the cause, Gaia received a whalloping blow to the stomach, and a multitude of thriving, diverse and vigorous animals, faced with ozone depletion and massive climatic changes, became extinct. Gaia herself, however, this living organism of which we are a part, recovered from this acute bout of colic. Some bone marrow or other genetic reserve was activated and a multitude of new life forms spilled out to fill in the hole in the biosphere.

We're not here because we out-witted the dinosaurs. We're not better nor more fit. We're just lucky, or, to rephrase an old moral adage, "There, with the dinosaurs, but for grace of God go we -- and there we may yet go." We are the living microcosmos taking new forms; we are the word of God re-phrasing itself. We are not, nor can we ever know, the final word.

Furthermore, evidence is accumulating from studies as varied as those of non-equilibrium chemistry to the biology of the Great Barrier Reef that the whole system, the whole organism, is not balanced in the sense that a steady-state or equilibrium system is. Gaia is more like a runner, tipped forward and slightly off balance, or like a developing embryo, not staying the same, but growing, changing, being "alive" in the full sense of that word. It is not only like an embryo: it is an embryo. The "balance of nature" takes on a whole new meaning in this context.

What does this mean for us? In the first place, from a personal point of view, I find the evidence that I am part of a larger evolving organism both exhilarating and humbling. Humbling because it is quite clear that Gaia does not need humans to survive; we could go the way of the dinosaurs and, as long as the essential bacteria were around, the homeostatic mechanisms would adjust. Exhilarating because whether our primary function in the global organism is merely to serve as a niche for anaerobic organisms in our intestines or whether we are the evolving brain of this whole enterprise, as unaware of our global thoughts as our individual brain cells are of us, we have a place here. This is our home. This is not a "space-ship earth" which we ride through empty space, mulling over our existential loneliness. The kind of humourless misanthropy that some so-called animal lovers or environmental activists generate -- the idea that people do not belong in Gaia -- has no place here. We belong here as much as (no more, no less than) the bacteria in the salt marshes and the prairie dogs on the plains.

At the same time, if the earth is a global organism, then we would expect her to consist of organs and organ systems like any other living animal. Some of those organs may be vital to her survival; at this point we're not sure which ones. Where are the "kidneys" that control the sea's salinity? Where do the detoxifying liver functions reside? Where are the crucial sites of respiration? We're a long way from being certain. Based on current research we are beginning to suspect that if, in our ignorance and arrogance, we destroy rain forests or intensively farm and pollute our continental shelves or build suburbs on our marshlands, the global "immune system" must surely get rid of us -- or Gaia will die.

Furthermore, as humans become an increasingly larger component of the earth's biomass, and as we consciously interfere with various body systems, we are acting as if our brains were to consciously take over all of our "unconscious" bodily functions -- respiration, digestion, regulation of trace minerals, and so on. As we take over those functions, we'd better make sure we know what we are doing. Right now, with all our child-like fascination with biotechnology and nuclear power, we toddle around the universe as if it were a laboratory outside of ourselves, carrying out potentially fatal experiments on the fetus of which we are a part.

Because of this global inter-connectedness, we can select just about any problem as a portal of entry and we find ourselves climbing up and down stairways that lead into other stairways that lead into still others, as if we were living inside one of those labyrinthine drawings by Esher or a Bach keyboard invention.

In many parts of the Third World, forests have been destroyed for firewood, resulting in land erosion and the loss of farmland. People in those parts of the world may spend as much time searching for fuel wood as they do on any other activity, but still have barely enough fuel to eat one hot meal per day. Is this a food problem? An agricultural problem? An energy problem? A population problem?

The temptation for North Americans is to treat the problems that face us in component parts, so that we can relegate the various parts to "experts". Thus we introduce new varieties of agricultural production without regard to the energy inputs required. So we remedy the next step by pouring in more fossil fuel or nuclear energy. But if every nation used as much oil per head in agriculture as the U.S., world oil reserves would be bankrupted within a dozen years, and the costs of such a short-sighted policy in acid rain, climatic change, and human destruction, we are only now beginning to realize. The nuclear option, on the other hand, requires that we guarantee a stable and peaceful society, and an earthquake-and-volcano-free earth for a hundred times longer than we've had human civilisation to date.

At the same time, back on the tropical farm, people are caught off-guard by the rising fuel prices; men go to the city to find extra work to help pay for the new off-farm inputs required to run the farm, and women stay behind with all the responsibility but none of the power or education they require to get the job done right. And more people leave the farm for the city. And there really are no jobs in the city, and the men are ashamed to go home with no money and take small comforts where they can, and AIDS spreads across the map. And agricultural land is further concentrated into fewer and fewer hands so it can be used to grow export crops to send to America to make money to pay for oil to run the farms. And our tropical "ally" asks for, and receives, extra military aid in order to keep its populations in line while it tries to cut its social programs for the displaced farmers in order to fit into IMF guidelines.

We could begin to describe similar webs of connectedness between North American hamburger eating habits, the destruction of the Brazilian rain forest and Third World military spending, or the entanglements of institutional racism against native peoples in Canada, massive destruction of Canadian forests, and the diapering habits of new parents in New York City. Or psychological problems of pets, carnivorous urban diets, environmental degradation secondary to agricultural production, and food safety issues.

This web-like nature of the world's biological and social systems is, at first glance, depressing. No matter what we tackle, we're caught in the tangles of the universal Black Widow.

Yet it is precisely because the earth is Gaia, an organism, like a huge, living, pliable 3-D puzzle, that these problems become manageable. We don't have to tackle all the problems head-on; if we only take on one serious problem, we've opened the door into the fun house. If we then change the shape of one small piece of that puzzle, we'll find that the picture is alive, that many of the other pieces -- with some extra prodding perhaps -- will change their shape to accommodate the newcomer. The words of Edmund Burke, spoken in another context, are most appropriate here, that "Nobody made a greater mistake than he who did nothing because he could do only a little".

A good local program of recycling and composting may not only stimulate other communities to do the same, but decreases urban pressures on wildlife preserves and conservation areas (by decreasing the need for landfill sites), encourages market gardening to accommodate the compost, decreases dependence on industrially produced and shipped vegetables (and thus decreases at the very least transport-related fossil fuel use), and, most importantly, gets people thinking about the earth's living cycles, its resilience and its limitations. Every bit of paper or metal or plastic recycled is important. Every compost heap is a cause for biospheric celebration.

The answers to the big problems will be small and multiple and diverse, tuned to local conditions: there is no one big answer to the pollution or the energy problems. In fact, the big answers are themselves often the biggest problems. Because of the earth's inter-connectedness, and because of its non-equilibrium balance, even small perturbations, if they are holistic rather than reductionist, and if they are appropriately placed and timed, carry with them a ripple effect, and the possibility of hope. Real hope is in the accumulation of many small personal and community actions.

We do need to be aware that real progress in implementing sustainable ways of living on this planet will involve a great deal more scientific carefulness that we have heretofore demonstrated. When dealing with any biological systems, we can never say for certain, for any given individual, whether a particular practice will be beneficial or detrimental. Epidemiological and ecological studies deal with probabilities, trends fringed with uncertainty, like boats with ripples of waves cresting away from them. Some scientists have in fact argued that this uncertainty is inherent in reality, that it is not simply a function of our incomplete knowledge. Indeed, probably the most commonly accepted truism among scientists today is that we can prove that something is not true, but we can never be absolutely sure that what we think is true, is really true.

The only reasonable way to proceed in this context of radical uncertainty is by means of a feedback loop system, the same way Gaia herself operates. Thus every technological interference, every health program, every development program, every re-cycling and suburban development program, should be designed and implemented as if it were a scientific experiment. The ecological impact studies that are sometimes carried out before, say, a dam is built, should only be the beginning. The implementation of the dam-building, if it is deemed appropriate, should be done in such a fashion that all the ecological ramifications of the actual dam-building can be measured, and the building process itself altered to suit the new data as it comes in. A program to control *Salmonella* in chickens or to build a new subdivision should be done the same, careful way.

Ultimately, the global problems we struggle with are all faces of the same dark angel: how can we live well and with dignity on this planet in the brief time we have been given.

None of us will, ultimately, save the world, but in caring for the earth and all that lives within it, and all the rocks and rivers which are the bones and sinews of Gaia, we may continue to grow with her, and not be cast aside as another of God's failed experiments.

There is a temptation, when looking for larger perspectives, to play that children's game: David Waltner-Toews, Maple Street, Guelph, Wellington County, Ontario, Canada, North America, Western Hemisphere, World, Solar System, Milky Way, Universe. . . If we move out into that vast, still darkness far enough, we may get a sense of the rhythms of an even larger life force. From the Big Bang of infinitely dense matter to our present state and back to the collapse into a single point may all be one respiration in the alveolus of the Great Being.

The danger in moving too far away from earth, however, is that we begin to feel lost again, alone among the stars, just when we were beginning to feel at home. The vision of life on earth which I like best, which I think is the most appropriate, proportionate to ourselves and our sense of being, comes to us from the pen of cancer researcher and physician, Dr. Lewis Thomas:

"The most beautiful object I have ever seen in a photograph, in all my life, is the planet Earth seen from the distance of the moon, hanging there in space, obviously alive. Although it seems at first glance to be made up of innumerable separate species of living things, on closer examination every one of its working parts, including us, is interdependently connected to all the other working parts. . . To put it another way, it is an organism. It came alive, I shall guess, 3.8 billion years ago today, and I wish it a happy birthday and a long life ahead, for our children and their grandchildren and theirs and theirs."

This is the real shape of earth, its only shape, and therefore its perfect shape. Gaia is the object of our love, and of our goodness. If we are to survive, it can be nothing less. And if we do not survive, I would still contend that it will have been better to have loved this planet -- richer, more exciting, *better* in the moral sense -- and then to have lost it, than never to have loved at all.

THE MAN IN THE CAGE

During a recent two-year stint as a veterinarian in Yogyakarta, Java, I sometimes found the density of my human surroundings to be unbearable. I would then brave the madhouse, crowded roads for an hour's drive up into the remotest canyon of the nearest volcano, Mount Merapi, and look for a spot that hadn't been claimed by six Boy Scout troops for the weekend, a few square yards where I could just breathe the air for a while. If I closed my eyes, I could even imagine that I was alone, that those village kids weren't waiting for me to open my eyes so they could sell me Coke. A little peace and quiet to do some of my most creative thinking -- about such topics as the virtues of crowding.

A friend of ours who lived in Yogyakarta hailed from the Yukon. Her living space in Java consisted of a small room squeezed between a garage and an English-language teaching institute. There was barely room for a bed, which was snug against the brick wall of the garage, and a couple of chairs. She bought her meals at a *warung* -- a food stall the size of a Canadian bathroom -- or from one of the myriad mobile street vendors who are common throughout Java. One evening, she had a couple of friends over, and they were talking about the compression of personal space that hits one upon entering Indonesian culture. In the middle of the conversation, the brick wall suddenly bulged, crumbled over onto the bed, and the front end of a car pushed its way into her room. No one was seriously injured though our friend sustained a few bruises on her legs where the bed had attacked her. An Indonesian in such a situation would brush herself off and continue as if nothing remarkable had occurred. Our friend, on the other hand, was too flabbergasted to respond. For her, the Yukon would never be the same.

A few weeks later, a team of workmen invaded our own house, fixing the places in the clay-tiled roof where monsoon rains leaked through, putting screens on the windows, unplugging the Western-style toilet ("It's because you use tissue," we were told disapprovingly), painting the walls, adding all the luxuries those annoying Westerners demand when they rent a house. The workers came every day for 10 days, and my wife became increasingly short-tempered. If they didn't water down the paint so much, they wouldn't have to paint the wall five times to get it white. And yes, they would have to put latches on the insides of the glass windows so that they could be opened, or else what was the point of the screens? (Indeed, they might have asked, what *was* the point?)

She was on the verge of a major fit one day when she sat down with one of the women who had been in the car-invaded room. "You're upset because you identify the limits of your house with the limits of your personal space," said our friend, somewhat accusingly. In North America, it seems perfectly reasonable to think of one's home as a kind of personal refuge not to be invaded at will by large groups of strangers. In Indonesia, such privacy has become a kind of selfishness. How could we not want the warm bodies of other people pressing around us continually? Were we misanthropists?

When I first arrived in Indonesia, I was overwhelmed by the sensory onslaught: the streets crowded with pedestrians, bicycles, motorbikes, minibuses, 2 or 3 people to a bicycle, 3 or 4 to a motorbike, 15 to a small van built for 8. It looked as if two-thirds of the population was under the age of 15. Even with the best possible birth control program in the world -- something, for Gaia's sake, devoutly to be wished for -- it's going to get worse, I thought, before it gets better. "Worse, better": a white man's bias right up front. The Western response to population pressures is to get vasectomies and tubal ligations to create fewer people and expect instant results (space, greenery, etc). The response in other parts of the world seems to be to adjust personal space. Peeople get used to having others around at closer quarters; they redefine their idea of privacy.

Various images come to mind: a very dirty, raggedly dressed man asleep on the sidewalk in Yogyakarta, his body moving to the rhythms of an obviously sexual dream. The crowds passed by, deliberately oblivious. He might as well have been in the privacy of a house. Or the farmer hanging his bum over the canal beside the road, watching me drive by in my Land Cruiser. This is normal, right? So why did I fuss and feel offended by it?

And yet, no matter how much I rationalize, how hard I try to retreat into a kind of critical mysticism, distancing myself within myself, I can't say I would like to sleep with several other men in the same bed, in a hot room with the windows closed (to keep out the disease-bringing cool breezes) and the lights on (to keep away Allah knows what). Am I in fact an evolutionary throwback, a maladapted dinosaur from a world that will never, despite all my wishful, bucolic thinking, exist again?

In a circuitous way, the cultural perception of personal space is important to our understanding of animal rights, of animal suffering, of animals in cages. There is a dairy farm in the city of Jakarta, in the shadow of clean-looking concrete skyscrapers. Narrow concrete walkways lead down between mud-plastered, whitewashed brick houses, along large, open sewers, and past apparently makeshift walls of corrugated metal and bamboo. In places, the sidewalks change to mud paths, skirted by plots of elephant grass or piles of rotting garbage being picked over by chickens, ducks and scavenging junk vendors. If you pull back a two-yard-high bamboo gate, you will see a dozen sleek, fat, black-and-white Holstein cows lined up in two neat rows along both sides of a clean cement-floored barn.

The farm has been here since the time of the Dutch, passed on from father to son, as the shantytowns of the city have sprawled up around it. The manure gurgles out the back of the open-walled barn into a huge, soupy pool not much different from some of the city's sewers. There, it is dried and sold in potato sacks for about 50 cents each. The cows are milked out into a pail. An old soup can is used to scoop the milk out of the pail and into two-or four-litre bottles (through a cloth filter to keep out the flies). It is then carried by bicycle or motorbike to milk-collection centres. Ultimately, much of *it* is dried too, and then has to compete with powdered milk dumped on the international market by more affluent nations.

The cows on these farms have never seen green pastures. They live in a closed ecological system that, among other things, cycles livers parasites out through the manure onto the plots of elephant grass, where they pass through snails, develop into a stage that is infective to cattle and return to the barn in armloads of freshly cut, hand-carried grass. All nicely balanced. The cattle are as healthy as any I have seen in Canada. And they are trapped. The only way out is on a meat hook. Is this an abuse of animals' rights? Should not these cows, philosophically ruminating though they may be, have access to rolling hills, fresh water, exercise? In another country, in another time, I might think this manner of keeping dairy cows to be an outrage, an infringement of natural animal rights. Is this case different? If so (and I think it is), what *makes* it different?

One difference, I think, is in the people who serve these animals. They, too, live in small concrete rooms that open onto narrow concrete walkways. They greet strangers with ready smiles and cups of tea and cakes. A mother sits on the walkway, spoon-feeding cassava porridge to the baby balanced on her hip. Other kids run around, making up street games; sounds are echoing everywhere, punctuated periodically by the calls to prayer or musical interludes blaring from the mosque's megaphone. Privacy, for people as well as for the animals they tend, is an internal matter; it is in your head.

At Christmas, my children received a couple of budgies from one of the neighbours. I dislike seeing animals in cages; so one day, after some minor prompting from the kids, I helped the birds out of their bamboo cage and into Matthew's bedroom. The female promptly flew to one wall, smacked her head against it, sagged to the floor, revived, flew to the other wall, smacked her head against that and finally cowered behind a metal window grate. The male managed to locate the wicker trunk full of kids' toys, which he climbed over and attacked with his beak. If there is something I like even less than seeing animals in cages, it is seeing them suffer. Clearly, this newfound freedom produced such anxiety in the birds that the cage was preferable. Back in their cage, after a night of rest, they groomed each other and sang.

If I were inclined toward a totalitarian ideology, I might be tempted to pontificate on the dangers of too much freedom and on the happiness of home and hearth. But I do ponder how power-fully Nurture can alter -- can, in fact, warp -- Nature. The birds were unable to handle their freedom because they had been bred and raised in cages. One cannot undo that kind of warping -- the kinds of warping we have inculcated into our agricultural animals over thousands of years -- by simply opening a few doors. But in a world growing more and more crowded, is it warping or sound prepara-tion to learn to live in cramped surroundings? History is full of examples of nature-warping, from our genetic selection and rearing of cattle and dogs to garden roses and caged birds. By what criteria do we call some of this warping and some of it adaptation? Who is right, the vasectomized North American who sits at the beach, watching the waves roll in, seeking inner peace through the contem-plation of nature, or the crowd of Indonesian students coming towards him, not wishing to see the poor soul have to sit by his lonely self with no one to talk to? I don't think I'm being devious by saying: they are both right, and our salvation will come through an integration, a Gandhian-type, dialectical learning from each other.

A number of years ago, there was a celebrated animal-rights case in Ontario involving the solitary confinement of a gorilla for a medical experiment. It seemed obvious to me that the treatment of the gorilla was cruel. What was not obvious was how to define that cruelty without sounding sentimental or Disney-esque or insensitive to the suffering of people in Ethiopia who might benefit from this medical research. (Always, of course, things are phrased this way, as if the suffering people of the world will benefit, not some big drug company or hospital corporation.) I finally decided that I was against the confinement of the gorilla because it was, scientifically, stupid to carry out an experiment on one animal. The results would have no statistical significance whatsoever. I knew, of course, that there were larger moral issues involved here, but no one was formulating them correctly, and somehow I couldn't get beyond that simple, morally righteous gut feeling of revulsion. Unfortunately, gut feelings seldom stand up well to criticism, though they may serve to energize more rational arguments.

A couple of years later, in Sumatra, I was standing before the pathetically small cage of an orangutan. He was sitting on the bare concrete, picking at himself out of boredom or depression. The gentleman beside me remarked how interesting this jungle creature was. Gazing at this orang-hutan (literally, man of the forest) imprisoned in a tiny cell for orang-kota (man of the city) to gawk at, I felt utterly helpless to transmit my dismay to either the man beside me or the man in the cage. I could identify with the rusty-haired man of the forest; I could feel the cruelty to him in my bones. But how could I communicate that feeling without reference to my ideas of privacy and personal space, ideas that are so culturally conditioned? And how was this caging different from the "caging" of the dairy cows in Jakarta or, for that matter, from the "caging" of the man standing beside me?

At the risk of attempting to answer from abstract principles a question that can, like all the great questions of life, be answered only by some sort of experiential integration, I'd like to suggest a possible path out of this maze of images. The answer, tentative as it may be, has to do both with my culturally conditioned sense of personal space and with the natural connectedness of all living things. The cruel treatment of animals, I would suggest, is that treatment which the perpetrator (zookeeper, farmer, pet owner) does not in some very real sense share with the animals. The zookeeper was not in there with the orangutan; the researcher did not live with his gorilla. Nor was there any sense, either in terms of material possibility or of empathetic feeling, that they ever would. A bettering of life, or a worsening of it, for the researcher of zookeeper bears no relationship, no connection, to the animal in his care. The city dairy farmers of Jakarta and their cattle, however, share the same cages, the same fate. The process of urbanization has not separated them from their animals; it has, rather thrown them even more closely together.

We, people and animals, should be crowding together, not separately. It shouldn't be us here in one part of town and the animals there in another, with the city expanding out into prime agricultural land, people complaining of animal smells, and farmers get pushed further and further to the periphery of society even as the demands made on them are greater and greater. We should get rid of all those anti-animal, keep-our-cities-pure zoning laws we have in North America and move our farm animals back into the cities so that people and animals can be with each other every day, cheek by jowl. When developers create one of their "housing estates", they should include in their plans several small, probably mixed, farms, where milk cows, chickens, and pigs might be raised, as well as vegetables and forages. The people who run these farms could do so full time, as individuals, or as part of a franchise, or cooperatively; the possibilities are as diverse as the people who think of them. The shopping plaza down the street should include a small abattoir, where the pigs and chickens and bull calves could be slaughtered for food.

What would this apparently far-fetched idea accomplish? With this re-integration of urban housing and agricultural production people would be able to see where their food was coming from. We'd probably have less meat eating and more outright vegetarians. While we were crowding together, there would paradoxically be more social pressure to have less crowding, for animals as well as for people; the limits to human and animal population growth are much more apparent in Jakarta than in Toronto, at least in part because Torontonians have designed their city to make animal crowding invisible. Diseases, both foodborne illnesses such as salmonellosis and strictly animal-related diseases, would be less of a problem in such a decentralized system. (Epidemics of disease thrive on large, homogeneous populations). Animal waste, which is a major disposal/pollution problem for intensive agricultural units, can be composted and recycled in the smaller amounts produced by smaller farms. With more animals around, dogs and cats would not be expected to carry the full burden of urbanites' disjunction from nature (which results is all sorts of pathological pet-human "bonds").

Is there a potential down-side? I suppose so -- if we would view such a move as a move "back", and let our animal-management skills slip. A decentralized, urban-integrated agricultural system would quickly slip into subsistence farming, or Jakarta-style slums, if we pretended that it required less sophisticated management or less scientific understanding than the current system.

In order to implement such an urban-rural integration, we need to recognize the incredible naivete -- stupidity, in fact -- of allowing the price of agricultural land to be determined by market values. An acre of land will be of greater financial value on the open market as a car-producing factory or a housing development than as a farm. But the comparison is simple-minded and ludicrous. Food production is primary and long-term, the basis of all other activities in our society. Now -- and in a million years -- we can live quite well without the car factory, which is in fact a destructive activity. We cannot live without the production of food. They are not in any way comparable activities. Even valuing land based on the value of the food potentially produced from that land in perpetuity would not give a fair price, since food is by its very nature irreplaceable. In every case, farming and food producing activities must be recognized as basic to all other activities and given priority. Housing and factories can survive quite well on marginal, non-productive land.

We share a common destiny with the animals on this planet, and it is the denial of this fact that leads to so much cruelty toward other species. The human race is in the process, at least in many urbanizing parts of the world, of altering its concepts of personal space and socially acceptable closeness. Some animal-rights activists have argued that in crowding our domestic animals together, we are warping nature and causing suffering. There are obvious extreme cases in which this is true. But what we also need to realize is that, from a global point of view, we're in for some heavy crowding over the next several hundred years, whether we like it or not, and if we want to survive gracefully, we had better keep up the warping. It is not the crowding that is wrong, it is how we crowd.

If we start rezoning now and moving the animals into suburbs, maybe by the time my children are grown up, or their children, North Americans will have caught up to the Japanese in their ability to adjust to having other living beings in close proximity. Maybe just in time. And if, by some freak miracle, the world population drops dramatically and we find ourselves surrounded by vast expanses of rejuvenated greenery, we will not forget the animals we have created. Having lived together, we will know each other, and we will walk from our cages hand in claw with our fellow domesticated animals.

SALMONELLA: A BRIEF INTRODUCTION TO FOOD POISONING

One of the first documented outbreaks of *Salmonella* food poisoning took place in France, in 1818. Napoleon was out and the old aristocracy decided to live it up at the castle. Very classy. Fresh oysters right out of the local moat. A few days later, 17 of the party-goers were very sick: abdominal cramps, diarrhoea, nausea, vomiting, head-and-muscle aches. The partyers felt so rotten they probably wished they were dead. Two of them were granted their wish. Quickly, the others repented, drinking the chicken soup and flat ginger ale prescribed by the doctor. Everybody used the toilet a lot. The toilets flushed into the moat, just around the corner from where the chef (a Napoleonic loyalist, no doubt) was counting out oysters for the next royal feast. So are the mighty humbled, even today.

Every year, from June through November, the Centers for Disease Control in Atlanta and the Laboratory Centre for Disease Control in Ottawa receive reports of small, localized epidemics of "summer flu." Most do not differ substantially from that first reported outbreak of Salmonella food poisoning. Today, the vehicles of transmission are most likely to be such picnic items as chicken salad, devilled eggs, raw (unexpurgated) milk, homemade ice cream, or (we didn't know what it was) cannabis. Most often, the source is much less obvious than a contaminated castle moat. If it's milk, the farm which provided it may be, to all appearances, clean and well run; perhaps a three-week-old calf, just weaned as part of an early-weaning "modernization" program, was found dead one morning; or one cow had a bout of diarrhoea -- but that was last winter for Pete's sake. Salmonellae make a lie of the one-bug-one-drug theory of disease; it would be impossible to fulfil Koch's postulates of causation for the bugs. Sometimes they make you sick; sometimes they don't. They are a constant reminder that we live in a globally circulating bacterial soup, and that much of what we call disease is an imbalance, an inharmonious screech in an otherwise remarkably melodic global body.

There are now reported to be a couple of thousand serotypes and strains of Salmonellae. They are truly a cosmopolitan group, bearing such names as *S. Heidelberg, S. San Diego, S. Dublin, S. New Brunswick, S. Montevideo, S. Muenster . . .* A place without a *Salmonella* is a place where no one is looking. Salmonella organisms, it may be safely said, are everywhere. They are also capable, given the right set of circumstances, of wreaking just about any kind of havoc: severe, watery, blood-flecked diarrhoea, pneumonia, arthritis, and septicemia (blood poisoning) in foals, piglets and calves; meningitis and kidney infections in children; the aforementioned summer flu; abortion and diarrhoea in cows, horses and pigs.

Or they may simply hang around (as they did in the notorious Typhoid Mary) and *wait* to cause problems. Poultry often carry the organisms around on their feathers without showing any signs of the disease. Recently, an epidemic of salmonellosis in the United States and Great Britain was traced to eggs. This is not in itself unusual; sometimes the bacteria hang around on the shell waiting for an opportunity to enter (like when you wash off its naturally protective cover, or when you inexpertly crack a dirty shell against the bowl's edge). The bugs in this most recent epidemic, however, appeared to have been laid inside some of the eggs, which was unusual. In other animals, recovered adults may sequester them in the gall bladder or, as with horses (which lack a gall bladder), in some of the intestinal lymph nodes. Such animals may appear to be healthy while intermittently spewing their little microbial fishes into the environment of the farm. In 1984, more than 2700 human cases in Canada were traced to one teat in one apparently healthy cow in Prince Edward Island. Calves that survive the disease often do poorly. Looking at microscopic pictures of their intestines, one wonders how they manage to "do" at all. I suppose if one were scatologically inclined, one could conceivably describe them as "making do."

If people pick up an infection from, say, raw milk, where does the milk get it from? Although the organism may be shed in the milk in acute stages of the disease, a more likely source is, perish the thought, "the environment". Feed, water, fertilizers, horses, pigs, sheep, ducks, dogs -- anything, in fact, that has a warm, moist component -- may be contaminated. Pet the dog and milk the cow; if there's Salmonella around, you've probably just contaminated your milk. Pluck the chicken, trim her at the cutting board, pop her into the oven, pull her out, slice her up on the same cutting board with the same hands and voila, the summer flu.

While identifying which of the 2000-odd Salmonellae did the job may indeed may be helpful in tracing the source of an epidemic, or mapping host specificities, it may not be of much help in preventing the disease. Like the most durable of politicians, Salmonellae are opportunists. They may hang around for months, or years, before actually disrupting the community. On a well run farm, the organisms may be common, but the disease rare. On the other hand, wherever animals are crowded, trucked, bought, sold, over-heated, chilled, overfed, underfed, poorly fed, or just plain sick, a few carpetbagging, paramilitary Salmonellae can stomp in and just lay the place waste. One could draw a very tight analogy between how human societies are run and the influence of Neo-Nazi groups, but that might be belabouring the obvious. To say that Salmonellae cause disease may, in many cases, be like attributing deaths after an airline disaster to the ensuing fire, and exonerating the mechanical failure that led to the crash.

Treatment of Salmonella-associated diseases, as with other diseases of dis-harmony, poses some difficulties for technically oriented medical practice. Many of the organisms are now resistant to the usually available antibiotics, either because of prior antibacterial use on farms or in people. And in horses, antibiotic treatment can sometimes actually precipitate an attack of salmonellosis, as if the organisms, driven to the wall in a kind of intestinal Stalingrad, explode outward in an orgy of pathologic defiance.

Deep in your soft, organic heart, you already know the treatment I would (usually) recommend. A comfortable bed, caring friends, and the imbibing of appropriate clear liquids are not only comforts for humans fallen on hard times, but may help a calf weather a stormy gut as well.

The very best treatment, as we are fond of hearing, is prevention. Clean calf pens, fly control (Muscovy ducks are good for this), manure removal, washing and drying udders before milking, and proper sanitation of all utensils (as well as hands) used for feeding calves or milking cows are all helpful. While the immortal Bob Dylan may have resented the way Maggie made him scrub the floor, sanitation in and around the milkhouse is more than just another pretty idea. If Salmonella is present in the herd, the manure will be contaminated. Organic fertilizers have been shown to be a source of infection in parts of Europe. Before being spread around anywhere, it should be disinfected by mixing it with lime to a two per cent solution. Better yet, a researcher from Sweden has found that proper composting, in which the manure pile gets up to at least 55C for at least a week, can kill off the bugs. Farm animal management should be aimed at reducing stresses as much as possible, keeping animals comfortable and well fed.

Make absolutely sure that those newborns get their first colostrum. Some vaccines are in the offing, but given the present lack of understanding as to how Salmonellae do their dirty work, I wouldn't hold my breath. If a cow has diarrhoea, isolate her and don't use her milk.

If you like your milk and steaks raw on the farm, fine. Consume them fresh on the farm, but don't try to convince me. I already know the city-slicking bacteria in my gut don't get along with the country bacteria on your farm. I love organic, but I love my body better -- and if I find you giving raw milk to my children, I shall have to report you. Such middle-class decadence should be reserved for consenting adults.

If you're throwing a royal fête, by all means serve chicken salad, devilled eggs, homemade ice cream and a glass of milk. But, to take liberties with the words of the psalmist, keep your hands hot and soapy, the food clean and cold, and your heart, just to hedge your bets, pure.

POTBELLIED PIGS AND THE NATURAL ORDER

Some twenty years ago, when I was a callow young student of English literature at a small Mennonite college in Indiana, I had some friends who adopted a piglet as a pet. The animal made a pink and jovial, if hypochondriac, companion, trotting about their upstairs apartment as if he indeed had been bred for the high life of the urban captive. Unfortunately for my friends, their landlord in the apartment below was not as pleased as they with the clattering of tiny feet across a hardwood floor or the squealing of anticipated discomfort, and gave them the usual ultimatum: you or your pig. This being the late 1960s, when pigs were paraded out as presidential candidates and compared with policemen, it seemed a particularly piquant snub to the landlord that they packed their bags and moved out, pig and all. Not long after, they had one of the fine house-and-garden parties for which they were known. It was a pig-roast, richly festive and touched with sadness. In retrospect, I think that pig, despite his odd life, came to a happier and more honest end than many of the animals who have evolved with us.

Robert Desowitz, in a fascinating book on parasites and their people entitled *New Guinea Tapeworms and Jewish Grandmothers*, tells the story of how, after the Indonesians annexed the half of New Guinea they call Irian Jaya, some of the tribespeople there began to suffer from a strange affliction. The people affected would go into fits and sometimes throw themselves into the fire and be badly burned. An investigation revealed that the source of the problem was a pacification gift from the President of Indonesia -- pigs from the island of Bali. The pigs brought with them not only their innocent hams and the president's best wishes for an unrebellious life, but a parasite which in people can sometimes migrate to the brain and make a cyst there.

For most people in urban North America, far removed from survival needs and blood sacrifices, the contractual arrangement which recognizes the mutual dependence between people and the rest of nature, the one demanding mutual respect and payments due, is rarely reflected upon. We make nature our plaything and create the illusion that life costs nothing biologically. I cannot help but wonder, is North American fascination with Vietnamese potbellied pigs and other "third world" pets, such as parrots, monkeys and some snakes, a way of becoming friendly with the earth's diversity, or is it, more darkly, just another form of pillage? And what will be the cost? For biologically, there is always a cost.

I first saw the little, black, potbellied pigs of Southeast Asia while working in the islands of Indonesia, where they are called *babi cina* (literally, Chinese pig), which through a linguisto-political trick is rendered into English as "Bali pig". I don't imagine my wife will ever let me forget the day I leapt from our minivan in Bali with a camera to try to get my first picture of them as they scampered away into a field -- while she was bent over on the seat suffering from a near-death experience with food poisoning. Despite their fat, loosely folded skin, sway-backed bouncing run and sagging bellies, they were too smart and fast for this foreigner to catch on film. It is of course in the nature of visitors to see a tropical paradise such as Bali through post-card lenses.

The Balinese might describe them differently. Relatives of the domestic pig, descended from the wild boar, *Sus scrofa*, whose history as a food animal goes back, along with the dog, some 5000 years in China, the potbellies are members of a clan of hundreds of locally adapted breeds of pigs, bearded pigs, warty pigs, and babirusa scattered throughout south and east Asia. Selected over centuries, they grow up to be less than 100 pounds, about the right size for a family meal, so that the availability of refrigeration, to save the leftover meat or transport it to market, is not essential. They are rugged, scavenging omnivores, roaming the streets and fields look-ing for garbage to clean up. Like many farm animals in that part of the world, they appear to be wild, but if you actually tried to steal one, you would quickly discover that (like North American cats) owners and pigs know each other quite well. They are a no-maintenance-cost animal of the kind detested by multinational feed and animal genetics companies. From an energy conservation and ecological point of view, for the future of a crowded planet, they are an ideal animal, and an ideal source of food.

Like Wilbur, the pig in E.B. White's *Charlotte's Web*, they are animals of keen intelligence, which is not surprising given their scavenging abilities under difficult circumstances, as well as being lively, trainable, and, to some minds conditioned to view animals as post-card pictures or animated cartoons, cute.

Having seen them in their natural habitat, I was more than mildly surprised and disturbed to see one come in to our veterinary clinic at Guelph this fall suffering (ironically) from a gastrointestinal disorder as a result of an inappropriate, pampered North American diet. I was even more surprised to learn that there are more than 8000 of them kept as pets in the United States and that they fetched a price of $500 to $5000 or even higher.

I have a nightmare. I imagine a terrible conspiracy of the excessively wealthy white North Americans against the poor people of Bali. In this nightmare, the little critters are Disney-fied, if I might coin a word, which in North America is as close to sanctification as popular culture will allow. According to the Gospel of Mickey Mouse, we cannot eat Bambi and his friends of course, nor should anyone else. Having made the little pigs too cute to eat, we then look the other way as our compatriots -- the analogues of the mercantile armies of the old empires who followed the missionaries -- offer large, white, energy inefficient and ecologically destructive Amerocanadian pigs as a substitute to the Balinese. It's just a bad dream of course. It will never happen. But I worry just the same.

There is one essential truth in Darwin's discoveries that has yet to sink into our collective consciousness: we are all part of the natural order. Neither cute little potbellied pigs, nor ducks, nor rats, nor people nor cats are outside of the intricate natural physiological web of our living planet. When ducks die off because of human intrusions into wetlands, or chickadees flourish because of artificial bird feeders, or cats are hit by cars or whales die because of environmental toxins, the question we face is not one of what is natural versus what is "unnatural". Since the bounds of our experience define the bounds of what is natural, it is impossible for anything to be unnatural. The questions we face are: how can we balance the biological integrity of birds against that of cats and insects? How can we relate to potbellied pigs honestly?

These are value-laden ethical questions, bound to stir up trouble and anguish. What kind of world do we wish to have? Which kinds of animals do we value? We will all die, as will all the animals we live with -- as, indeed, will the planetary organism of which we are a part. Death is not the issue; death gives boundaries and urgency to a more important question: how can we most honourably live together before our deaths?

The little potbellied pigs of south China and Southeast Asia evolved over thousands of years to fit a particular socio-ecological niche. They are not dogs, nor cats, nor are they Wilbur, the fat white Yorkshire pig. Having evolved in the tropics with little hair covering their bodies, potbellied pigs need a warm sleeping environment (60-70 degrees F), and may dig into and shred their nests if uncomfortable. In fact, it is probably cruel to prevent them from engaging in their natural inclinations to dig in the dirt. On the other hand, they are like water buffaloes and Californians in that they do not sweat, and hence require shade and a cool pool in hot weather. Having evolved on a rough and ready diet of food scraps and coarse vegetation, the highly refined corn-based diet of North American fattening hogs, if used at all, should be supplemented with fresh vegetables, forages, and fruits. Having evolved as scavengers, however, they're not really fussy, and can poison themselves by eating plants like rhubarb leaves or lily of the valley.

In order to satisfy our "refined" surroundings, the male tusks need to be cut yearly, so we don't get hurt handling them. The hoofs might need trimming if the pigs don't get out and around enough. As well, the pigs need to be protected from people who might want to lift them by the front legs, dog-like, as this can dislocate their shoulders, or flash bulbs, which can frighten them. The female delights of sexual arousal every three weeks, may wear a bit thin on some owners and require reproductive control. Of course, they will need vaccinations for various diseases such as parvovirus, erysipelas, leptospirosis and some diarrhoeal agents.

The keen intelligence of the little potbellies has been honed in the struggle to survive in difficult circumstances. I am not surprised that they are affectionate, and can be toilet-trained if you are willing to take them out every four hours during the day. In the end, however, I cannot believe that it is a sign of respect to that intelligence, nor a credit to ours, to make those animals our playthings -- no matter how well we care for them.

Are we doing them a favour to take them out of their home environment and introduce them to the aches and pains of old age (10-15 years in a potbelly)? A quick death in the prime of life -- and as one whose father died suddenly and unexpectedly I do not say this lightly -- may be one of Nature's favours. What we do not like, of course, is that for some animals whose evolution has been closely intertwined with our own, we may be called upon to act as Nature's hand in this. We would just as soon pretend that death has nothing to do with us, which is why we eat meat but want to avoid the subject of slaughterhouses. We want to own pets, and preserve them from an honest death.

What it comes down to, then, is this: just a little respect, in life as in death.

William Youatt, in an 1855 treatise on *The Hog* tells the story of a gentleman from Caversham, who, having purchased two pigs at Reading market, had them conveyed home in a sack. The following morning, finding the pigs gone, he raised a hue and cry; that afternoon, he was apprised of a sighting of two pigs swimming across the Thames River near his home. A second sighting was reported near a crossroads, where the pigs were seen with their noses together, "as if in deep consultation". The destination of their journey turned out to be the farm from which they had been conveyed to the Reading market, a distance of some nine miles. The farmer, being an honest man, returned the pigs to the purchaser in Caversham. The pigs, being both intelligent and stubborn, repeated their homeward journey the following day. The story illustrates, we are told, the "great sagacity" of swine. We are not told the ending.

I confess that when I see the little Vietnamese potbellied pigs garlanded and leashed and pampered, I imagine them commandeering a leaky vessel and navigating the seven seas back to their tropical home. A hot place, yes, a place where it's man eat pig and pig eat scraps and they are unlikely to get ice-cream. It's a place where, even as they are being eaten -- indeed only as they are being eaten -- that they can help to give new life to the parasite *Taenia solium* and in so doing both repay a debt to nature for having been given life, and extract a cost from people for having taken life. It's home, then, and one of the few places left on earth where a small pig can still make an honest living.

ANIMAL RIGHTS: GAIA RIGHTS

The language and posturing of both the animal rights activists and the powerful exploiters against whom they labour are the creation of lawyers, and are caricatures of two basic truths. Nature is neither our friend (as those on the one extreme imply) nor our enemy (as those on the other extreme imply). Nature is, and we are part of it. To subdivide the natural world into moral categories based on some a priori system demonstrates a lack of respect for the world-in-itself. Yes, there are rights involved; for instance, the right of the carnivores to attack and kill their prey, the rights of the bacteria to recycle my body when I'm gone, as well as the rights of animals to behave "naturally" and to be free from suffering. I do not, however, respect those rights. I respect the animals and beings and entities, who with me are part of a greater created being, in and of themselves. The rights flow from that respect. And that, I would argue, is fundamentally different from arguing for or against animal rights, which, by focusing on a symptom only, are disrespectful to all of us.

I have trouble believing the people who fight against animal rights. These are the same technocrats who told us that the nuclear weapons have prevented another world war. They are masters at Orwellian doublespeak. More than twenty million people, most of them civilians, most of them in the Third World, have been killed in the Third World War, that proxy non-nuclear war fought by the "great" powers in Angola, Vietnam, Afghanistan, El Salvador and dozens of other neo-colonized countries. In the same way, millions of animals and living eco-organs within Gaia are suffering at our hands even as we speak of environmental cleanup and safe food.

I also have difficulty believing the animal rights defenders, however. They are taking the same tired old moral paradigms that we have applied step by step to men, women, slaves, other "races" -- though women of "other races" are still slaves in a large proportion of the world -- and now to animals. The logical framework for this way of thinking is fundamentally flawed. It is based on classifying nature into groups and then confusing the expedient metaphors (men, women, mammals,etc.) with nature itself. Nature is continuous and unclassified.

The application of the human biomedical paradigm -- which is a combination of ingenious natural classification schemes with moral classification schemes -- while saving many individuals at particular points in time, is resulting in an immense increase in human suffering overall. By saying that each human life is "beyond value" those who are rich and powerful in the industrialized West have managed to divert huge amounts of resources to saving a few. The necessary corollary to this is that in practice, ironically, those few lives are treated as being more valuable than millions of others in the Third World. As I am writing this, television is devoting many hours to talking about a dozen or two people who died in California as a result of a fire, and no time at all to the many hundreds who died at the same time as the result of an earthquake in India. Nor is this an anomaly. The war against Iraq, which killed hundreds of thousands of young people and children either through direct hits or post-war starvation, is widely regarded as a victory. Our moral considerations are consistently and fundamentally skewed. To assuage our guilt, we engage in vaccination programs to save the lives of millions of babies, only to turn the other way a few years later when they starve to death.

This same paradigm is used to save a few mammals that we find cute or necessary to our wellbeing, while allowing us to plunder the inherently wonderful creation around us.

Concerns for suffering in other animals -- not just in the artificial domestic animals we have created, nor the suffering of those animals in whose into whose eyes we so easily project our own suffering, but in all animals -- takes on a different meaning when considered in the context of a global, living being. Just as human rights are meaningless and destructive unless considered in perpetual tension with human responsibilities, so animal rights are meaningless and destructive unless they live in tension with what we might call "ecological responsibility". The suffering of individuals in the biosphere is like localized pain; it may not be life-threatening, but it is still pain, something to care for and pay attention to, and is a diagnostic warning that something isn't functioning right. When my kidney went into spasms around a lovely multi-spiked crystal in 1974, I would not have been much impressed by a doctor who advised me not to worry, the pain is only local. The language of respect can serve as a basis for definition of rights -- and limitation of those rights, within, say, an Animal Welfare Act, implemented by trained professionals. In this regard, then, those of us who care for the whole earth can keep company with the animal rights philosophers.

At the same time, the arguments for animal welfare no longer depend on anthropomorphism, or utilitarianism, or any other human-dependent moral schemes. We care for all the other members of this globe -- bacteria in the marshes as much as seals off the coast -- because we are all part of the same Gaia, just as my brain cares about my stomach and my toenails because they are part of me. The elevation of the earth to this moral status also provides limits to the application of rational moral arguments to non-human life. Ecology and biology are also relevant here -- which is not to say, simplistically, that what is natural must necessarily be good. This misses the point that everything that is, is natural by virtue of its being. Nevertheless we can say that the vigour and creative energy of the natural world is relevant to our ideas of what is good. Death is not the greatest evil in Gaia; death is an essential way for Gaia to recycle nutrients within herself. The questions relate to how we live, and how we die, not whether.

While species extinction has a hard time finding a moral home in the language of suffering and rights, we may view the daily extinction of plant and animal species as the removal of various bodily organs from Gaia. Many of them may not be essential: you can lose a few fingers and pieces of intestine and still survive. But it seems to me that the gratuitous lopping off of bodily organs without any idea as to what function they serve, or could be destined to serve in case of another cosmic accident, is a questionable medical practice.

The economic arguments sometimes used to justify the destruction of forests and marshlands begin to sound like those of a doctor caught making living by resecting healthy sections of intestine from people. "But I make a good living at it!" he might argue. I think we would advise him to find another way to make a living. So why do we tolerate it on a global scale? No developer should be allowed to fill in a marsh or cut down a tree; on a world scale, this should only be done if it can be demonstrated that the marsh represents an acute risk to human life and that there are no other ecologically acceptable solutions.

No forestry company should be given an acre more of land to cut from; they should be forced by law to recycle on the hundreds of thousands of acres we've given them already. If they don't want to farm trees on a sustainable basis, they should get out of the business. What would we say if farmers from Ontario invaded Manitoba saying, well, we haven't planted crops for a few years so we thought we'd harvest yours? That's what the lumber companies do. I am dismayed that unionized woodworkers allow themselves to be used as cannon fodder by management against native peoples and environmentalists. It is as if they had taken to heart Jonathan Swift's ideas about solving the Irish famine by eating children, skewering their own children for the sake of a company job today. I am also dismayed at the environmentalists, who, by focusing on saving the trees and the baby seals, rather than on seeking creative solutions to the issues of how people can live well (morally and economically) in relationship to the environment and each other, have chosen the easiest, most destructive and, in the long run least successful path to solving our most severe environmental problems.

The care of wildlife, and the preservation of habitat to prevent wildlife diseases takes on a new meaning. This is particularly true as we determine where, in fact, the vital organs on this planet really are. We should be vitally concerned that the research to make those determinations gets funded and is carried out, and that our knowledge of living animal systems is brought to bear on that research.

Granting native peoples full rights on the huge tracts of land which are rightfully theirs will, at the very least, buy us and our planet time until we come to our ecological senses. I have no illusions that native peoples are *necessarily* more (or less) responsible and ecologically conscious than anyone else (we have all, in truth, sinned). However, there are few enough of them and the lands they have claim to are so vast that, even given a worst-case scenario, they cannot possibly do as much harm as we are doing today.

What I am saying is this: that we should go beyond the legal languages of rights and welfare and implement practical measures based on global self-respect. If we respect each other -- if we respect ourselves as a global being -- then the necessary tension between individual rights and global responsibilities will not only be manageable, but a source of creative energy.

PART II:

GOATS

RUMEN AT THE TOP

When the primordial swamp hiccoughed the first amphibious life forms onto its shores, one of the little toadies decided to take a piece of the old home swamp along on his journey. I can think of no more logical reason for the existence of a cow, sheep, goat or reindeer. From an anatomical point of view, these animals are little more than large vats of swamp water stuck in various carriage models. The vat is called the rumen, the so-called first of four stomachs, and the animals themselves, sensibly enough, are called ruminants.

Camels, llamas, some leaf-eating monkeys and hippopotami are halfhearted ruminants whose stomachs have compartments, but they have made a definite break, anatomically speaking, from their boggy past. Elephants, horses, apes, rabbits and beavers have developed a kind of backward ruminant system, whereby the caecum, the large sac at the entrance to the colon -- serves as a fermenting barrel. Only the rabbit, however, is agile and humble enough to avail itself of the extra nutrients thereof, in an act that is best left to bathroom graffiti and scientific journals for description.

The nature of the ruminant's stomach system, and in particular the nature of the rumen itself, determines what feeds can be dangerous to the animal, what the nature of these dangers is and what remedies can be suggested.

If one avails oneself of a child's plastic stethoscope or, more cosily, simply applies one's ear to the fuzzy left flank of a cow or a goat, one can actually hear the rumen rumbling. Listen at the depression in the flank between the last rib and the hipbone. About one to three times per minute in a healthy cow, more often in a sheep or goat, a distant prairie storm thunders in from the fore of the animal, followed shortly by an echo from the aft. These sounds, more pleasing to some of us prairie kids than the sea in a shell, are the sounds of the muscular rumen walls and its internal folds and pillars contracting, washing the rumen fluid up and over the thick layer of food scum at its surface. This fluid is teeming with unicellular and bacterial life and, in fact, is the key to this whole marvellous system.

The sad truth is that although all animal life depends on green plants to trap the energy of the sun, no animals larger than bacteria are capable of digesting the most common form of stored plant energy: cellulose. Even termites depend on the bacteria in their guts to digest wood. Bacteria, it might be said, are priests in the temple of the sun god -- and workerpriests at that.

The rumen is very much a racially mixed, communal hot tub of bacteria and paramecia. There are not only cellulolytic (cellulose-digesting) bacteria but also populations of workers that specialize in digesting starches, sugars, protein, fat and urea. The entire balanced ecosystem is adapted to function optimally at a temperature of 102 to 104 degrees F, in the absence of oxygen, at a pH of 5.5 to 7 and in the presence of moderate amounts of fermentation products. Although there has been talk in scientific journals of using recombinant DNA techniques to alter the genetic makeup of rumen bacteria, they are tuned, in their natural state, to play their most harmonious digestive music on forage foods such as grass and hay.

Partially digested feed, fermentation products (the ruminant's prime source of energy, composed mostly of acetic, propionic and butyric acids) and dead bacteria spill over into the reticulum (the second stomach) -- a small, muscular organ with reticulated walls -- squeeze between the booklike leaves of the omasum (the third stomach) and finally enter the abomasum (the fourth stomach, comparable to our own), where the cow itself begins to digest its own food. In order to neutralize the acids produced by the bacteria and to keep the rumen comfortable, a cow will produce, every day, 22 to 42 gallons of jogger's juice: saliva laced with trace minerals and baking soda and with a pH of about 8.2 (which makes it a base and thus enables it to neutralize acidic fluids that have a pH below 7). In their fermentative excitement, the bacteria also produce about 330 gallons of gas per day, mostly methane and carbon dioxide, which the cow, if she is to remain functional, must belch up in a process referred to in polite circles as eructation. It is this process which some have suggested is contributing significantly to the buildup of the greenhouse gas methane in the environment. In principle, the people who say this are correct, but it seems to me that the role of cows, versus buffaloes, goats, and rice paddies needs to be clarified before we decide whom to shoot first, and whether we should deify Buffalo Bill as a patron saint in having reduced greenhouse gases.

With this complex, balanced system in mind, we begin to appreciate some of the potential problems to which ruminants are prone. One of the more spectacular veterinary disasters on record involved a British veterinarian who, in a fit of professional flair, lit a match at the mouth of an eructating cow. The resulting conflagration destroyed the entire barn. Most ruminant digestive problems are, however, more mundane.

Since the rumen is designed to handle forage, almost any other food taken in excess or introduced too quickly can cause serious problems. Overdoses of carbohydrate-rich foods, such as grains, apples, grapes, baker's dough, sugar beets, mangels and sour wet brewer's grains, can result in a rapid overproduction of acid in the rumen. This can throw the whole system off balance so rapidly that animals can go from looking drunk to looking (and even being) dead within a matter of hours.

If you catch your friendly farmyard ruminant with her nose in the grain and a sluggish, green smile on her lips, you will need to act fairly quickly to save her. Keep her up and walking around. Offer only small amounts of dry hay, ration her water intake, and dose her with the basic "I can't believe I ate the whole thing" remedy: a pound of baking soda (sodium bicarbonate) in two gallons of warm water should do for an overloaded cow, as will the same amount of milk of magnesia (magnesium hydroxide). A sheep or goat may come around with as little as eight ounces of milk of magnesia. Cow-sized doses of magnesium hydroxide should be available at feed stores or veterinary clinics; you would have to clean out your local pharmacy's entire supply in order to get a large enough dose from human formulations.

If your ruminant survives the initial engorgement episode, she may still develop chronic problems. Since the large amounts of acid in the rumen can kill off most of the productive inhabitants of the swamp, she becomes listless, does not eat and cannot digest her food. If you listen at her left flank, the thunder is gone; a bit of post-storm dripping and splashing remains, perhaps, but nothing like the abdominal rumblings of a healthy animal. The only good remedy is to send some hardy new bacterial immigrants in to repopulate the swamp. These can be enlisted either by going to the nearest abattoir and signing up for a pail of rumen juice or by simply siphoning some out of a friendly neighbouring ruminant. The juice is then pumped through a stomach tube or poured from a pop bottle into the listless, hungover cow.

Another side effect of acute carbohydrate engorgement is that the rumen wall is damaged (ulcerated), allowing some of the rumen bacteria to leak through into the blood. After the blood is filtered through the liver, any bacteria having a joyride are attacked by white cells and walled off into abscesses. A similar process can occur in animals that are chronically subjected to high-class diets; liver abscesses are common in calves or sheep raised in feedlots. Feedlot owners gamble that animals on a "hot" diet will grow faster, and they are willing to sacrifice a few livers for the extra pounds of meat at slaughter. Occasionally, however, one of those liver abscesses will rupture into the bloodstream, rapidly killing the animal, in which case the gamble does not pay off. As in people, living the high life can lead to ulcers, bad livers and a chronic dependency on antacids.

A piece of equipment that is essential for handling ruminant digestive emergencies is a length of several feet of soft rubber hose (a garden hose will do in a pinch) with one end rounded off. A piece of metal pipe, slightly larger in diameter than the hose, can be set into the animal's mouth in order to discourage her from biting through your valuable new tool, and a slathering of vaseline or mineral oil will ease the tube's insertion through your bovine friend's oral orifice and down her throat.

While many of a ruminant's digestive difficulties can be traced to acid indigestion, others, some of them fatal, are related to gas production. If the continuously produced rumen gas cannot, for some reason, escape on the sweet wings of a bovine belch, it will build up inside, bulging the rumen wall out the left flank. If left unchecked, it can cut off the general circulation and kill the animal. The father of this fatal gaseous pregnancy can be something as simple as a potato or an apple lodged in the throat. I confess I have occasionally pondered the possible bovine origins of the political profession, and the unhappy fate of some of our politicians if they kept their mouths shut too long. This consideration allows me to be a little more forgiving of some of their excesses.

The rubber hose, well lubricated, can be used to gently nudge the obstacle down into the rumen. If the bloat is well advanced and the cow or goat is on the verge of collapse, a quick stab with a clean knife or large trochar into the bulging left flank can bring immediate symptomatic relief. This procedure will give you more time to work on removing the offending obstacle but should be accompanied by a shot of penicillin in the hip to guard against infection.

Any cow, sheep or goat with such an obstruction in her throat will slobber a lot, since the same door that keeps the gas in also keeps the beast's voluminous saliva out. This combination of fat, gassy gut and slobbering mouth can help you determine which of several pathological states your animal is in. With rabies, for example, you are likely to see more slobbering than bloat, since the problem relates to an inability to swallow. The rabid beast is also likely to be slightly wobbly in the hind end. Occasionally, and for no apparent reason, sheep or cattle on a high-grain diet will develop a free gas bloat. This will be relieved by the passage of a stomach tube.

Foamy bloat is another matter. A good, munchy dose of alfalfa will cause the rumen bacteria to let out their gas in a continuous flow of stiffwalled bubbles. For all I know, the bacterial kids are simply having the time of their lives in the old hot tub. Unfortunately, the animal is unable to eructate these bubbles; neither is the stomach tube by itself nor a stab in the side of any use in this case. A good dose of mineral oil or dioctyl sodium sulfosuccinate (DOSS), available commercially in many stores, will break down the foam and allow your grateful friend to burp up her gas. If you have a ruminant given to free gas buildup, or to whom you have administered a dose of mineral oil to encourage belching, tie a stick crossways in her mouth. This forces her to keep her mouth and throat moving, thus letting out the offensive gas.

Some feed is dangerous to the ruminant not because of the structure of the ruminant stomach but because of the feed's inherent nature. Take a nail, for instance. Since cattle explore with their tongues, much like children, any piece of junk of appropriate size is likely to end up going down the hatch. A nail will drop right down through the rumen into the second stomach, the reticulum, which in a fit of righteous rage will contract around it and stab itself. If the animal is lucky, the nail will be walled off into a small abscess, and that will be the end of the matter. If not, the abscess may form near a nerve and interfere with the normal stomach movements. If she is Irish, the nail may wander over to the heart and, like any passionately held, stiff-as-steel ideology, pierce her to the quick. Many feed stores and vet clinics sell large magnets that can be dropped into your ruminant junk collector. These are meant to encourage wires and nails and such to stay in the stomach instead of wandering off on some death-dealing journey. Magnets probably function better if administered before the nail is eaten.

Cattle turned on to lush pasture in the late fall sometimes develop a crackling, wheezing pneumonia. This was traditionally called bovine asthma, fog fever, emphysema and a host of other names, and is now most often referred to as atypical interstitial pneumonia (AIP), reflecting our continued ignorance as to why it occurs. The affected cattle may have emphysema so badly that not only do the alveoli (the little pink saclike structures that comprise the lung) rupture, but the gas from the lung actually escapes and is pushed up under the skin over the shoulders. If you pass your hand over this area, you can feel it crackling like that bubbly packing plastic. This appears to be an allergic reaction to something in the pasture and is a real danger if you are taking over an old property and using its pastures for the first time in many years. In this case, it is better to ration the time on pasture, keeping your eyes open for problems. Steroids, antihistamines and atropine (obtained from belladonna) may provide some relief once a cow is sick, but nothing works really well.

Mouldy sweet clover hay, bracken fern and brassica plants such as rape and kale can, for different reasons, cause anaemia and bleeding disorders in ruminants if they are eaten continuously or in large amounts. Also, as the Cuban government discovered a few years ago, a diet of molasses, urea and sugar-cane pulp can result in soft spots in the brain (polioencephalomalacia). As this diet sounds remarkably similar to the kind of fare to which many North American children are subjected, it makes one wonder if there has been raised a whole generation with soft brains as well as soft teeth, and if this may be the real root of some of our present political insanities.

The list of poisonous or potentially poisonous plants is endless and, perhaps, pointless. A little grain, a little candy, or even, in many instances, a little poison, will not unduly upset a cow or sheep or goat. The rumen is, when all is said and done, quite a resilient little ecosystem.

Variations on one basic rule should suffice for most situations: hay for the hungry, grass for the greedy, forage for the famished. Silage may be viewed as a modified forage, and ruminants can adapt to it over time just as a person can adapt to a diet of sauerkraut. But be advised that such adaptation alters the delicate balance of one's intestinal ecology. Some feed additives, called ionophores, may alter the rumen microflora to utilize silage more efficiently, but these sorts of dietary and rumenary manipulations really are not suitable for smallscale farming.

Any new feed should be introduced gradually, for fear of upsetting the rumenal Yin-Yang. Keep a careful record of your animals, including feed changes and incidence of disease. Then, when planning next year's menu, ruminate, and you will have some hard evidence to go on. Your ruminant may forgive your menu planning if you are naive, but not if you are stupid enough to repeat past mistakes. She may forgive the blind, but not the oblivious. If she does not like the food, you can be sure that she will let you know. In the immortal words of Dr. O.M. Radostits, addressed to a class of green vets armed with needle in one hand and textbook in the other: "You'll miss more for not lookin' than for not knowin'." That is as true for feeding barnyard ruminants as it is for life in general.

Ruminants have been much maligned by some environmentalists in recent years, in some cases justifiably. One statement, however, which I have heard repeated in a couple of settings goes something like this: you can produce 350 lbs. of soybeans and 265 pounds of rice on the same acre as you can produce 82 lbs. of dairy products and 20 lbs. of beef. Standing at the edge of Saskatoon, looking out over the prairie grasslands, I wonder about this. I confess that I remain to be convinced that tearing up prairie range pastures to make rice paddies would be progress.

SOUP AND THE ART OF GOAT SELECTION

When buying goats, as when buying groceries, it is advisable to be armed with a shopping list, so as not to arrive home with an armful of unnecessary bargains and no enthusiasm left to care properly for the creatures. Browse through the appropriate journals. Read a few introductory books on goat keeping, and, most importantly, visit and talk with people who already own goats. If you don't know anyone, see if there is a goat exhibition at your local agricultural fair, or check the classifieds in your community newspaper. Be relentless in your pursuit of information. Be wary of schmaltzy testimonials.

Included in your preliminary investigations should be a consideration of your facilities availability of feed, housing, fencing. Sit on this information for a while. Take a cue from the intelligent animal you are about to share your life with: ruminate. When you have digested the information and familiarized yourself with the kinds of goats that are available in your community, be warned of this one last thing: the learning of books, journals and well-meaning homilies such as this are but a pale facsimile of the real knowledge of raising goats. In caring for your first goat, as in acquiring any substantial knowledge, you will make mistakes. You will sleep better at night if the mistakes are made on animals of less than extraordinary financial worth.

It is unlikely that you will find a goat which is both an excellent milker and an excellent meat producer. In the words of Aristotle, "What Nature takes away from one place she puts on in another." While this holds true for meat and milk, it is not always true for other characteristics: the congenital absence of horns, for instance, does not betoken a displacement of horn energy into, say, the sex organs. The opposite may, in fact, be true, and polled stock (that is, stock bred not to have horns) may have fertility problems. A comparison of slow reproductive rates in the heavily polled populations of industrialized countries with the higher rates in countries where pollsters are less prevalent might lead one to believe that this might be a newly discovered general rule of nature. This, in turn, suggests some interesting possibilities for population control which should be pursued.

Of goats available in North America, Saanens have the reputation for being the heaviest milkers and Nubians are noted for putting on flesh quickly, but individual animals vary a great deal, and the Toggenburg mama you look at may be a top milker or the La Mancha kid a fast grower. Whatever you buy, have a checklist of desirable physical characteristics along, just to make sure you don't forget anything. Are her eyes bright and alert, her lips muscular, her neck clean-cut? Does she have a deep chest and a full, but not sagging, belly? These are all traits you want. A healthy goat has clean, supple skin. The slope from her hips down to her tail should not be too steep, and she should stand squarely on all four feet. Pick up her feet; are they trimmed and clean? If she is in milk, let the owner demonstrate milking for you, just to see how well she stands, or if she is a kicker. Feel her udder. A good udder is soft and pliable: no lumps, no extra teats (although these can be trimmed off in young stock) and no asymmetry. If you're hand milking, ensure that the teats aren't too long or too short for your hands. Teats that point out to the side are good for feeding cats but that's all; they're asking to be kicked and damaged. Neither do you want an udder that doubles as a barn sweeper.

Check her skin for lice, and, before buying, have a vet clinic check her stool for parasite eggs. Both lice and worms can be destroyed, but better to treat them at the seller's than to bring them home to your place. Find out exactly what she's being fed so that you don't, in a sudden outburst of romantic love, increase her daily dose of grain and give her a fatal case of indigestion.

If you are buying young stock, look for the clean-cut, lanky adolescents. They fill out much more quickly and efficiently than do the stout, mature-looking kids.

Avoid a mature horned goat unless you really, deep down in your aesthetic belly, need those horns. Kids with horns can be disbudded; taking the horns off a mature ram can be a veterinarian's nightmare. There is very little room between the base of a goat's horn and the top of his brain, and one doesn't wish to interfere with the brain, there being little enough to begin with.

For the starting goat-steader, a couple of inexpensive, bred female goatlings of a breed locally available would be the best buy. In this way, the goats can get accustomed to you and yours before they kid, you can make your mistakes on inexpensive animals, and sires of the same breed will be available if you wish to upgrade your "flock" in future years. With a generation interval of only a year, goats can be upgraded quickly by breeding back to high quality sires. Finally, since goats are gregarious animals, you may have better fortunes with two animals than with one.

Hybrid vigour, the increased hardiness, vitality and growth rate often seen in crossbred animals, can be taken advantage of if you have, say, a good milker but you want meaty kids (I shall refrain from drawing any human parallels on that one). One animal geneticist informed me that some owners are obtaining good meat carcasses from a Nubian buck bred to local or non-Nubian females.

Since male kids are often destined for the stew pot and females more often for the milk house, it would be lovely to be able to decide in advance the sex of the kids so that you could choose your sire accordingly. For all the work being done on chemical tests and electron microscopic examination of sperm tails, no reliable indicators are yet available, and we are left with little but folk advice. Some of this advice, such as that offered by Aristotle, stretches the limits of credibility, but offers at least the comfortable illusion that one is doing something. It is the same advice I would give people who would prefer offspring of one sexual type or another; in fact, it is the only advice I think they should ever get.

> "Some give birth to females, others to males, and the difference is due to the waters they drink (some waters are productive of females, some of males) and to sires in the same way. If copulation takes place while the north winds are blowing, they tend to produce males, if south winds, females. Female-bearing animals may change over to become male-bearing: they must face north during their intercourse."

In closing, then, we might say that, in buying goats as in buying soup, a Heinz 57 will provide adequate sustenance for the beginner, provided one has carefully read the label.

IT MAY BE A EUPHEMISM TO YOU

"It may be sh*t to you, but it's my bread and butter," is a saying that is sometimes ascribed to parasitologists, but could be spoken with great force and conviction by any practising farm veterinarian. Many euphemisms have been used to describe it, but as one who has spent many hours with his arm immersed in a cow's colon, or peering at stool samples through a microscope, I fail to see how altering the language can in any way alter the reality. It smells the same in a shirt and tie as in the gutter. However, in deference to those who know neither the changing of diapers nor the delights of the honeywagon, I shall refer to it by its respectable names within the confines of this article, or, where those fail, fall back on the capitalized, gender and species neutral pronoun IT.

The modern, Western industrialized urban aversion to IT may be, following Jean-Paul Sartre's reasoning, a complication of a more basic existential nausea. Nevertheless, other societies have managed to cope with ITs daily close presence in ways more creative than simple retching. Some cultures have had gods associated with IT. The ancient Greek hero Ajax, whose name came to be associated with the privy, has been traced via Jupiter, "the father of us all" (Ovid) to Stercutius, the god who invented manuring the fields and who was celebrated for his good husbandry. The Romans (Crepitus) and the ancient Egyptians (le Pet) even included personifications of flatulence -- seriously or not -- in their pantheons of gods. Sometimes love, dung and fertility have become confused in the public eye, as in the close connection of Cloacina, the Roman sewer god, with Venus, or in the ancient Mexican goddess Tlacolquani, "eater of ordure," who also presided over loves and carnal pleasures. The childish fascination with excrement which so fascinated Freud, would appear to have deeper roots than just bad habit or mineral deficiency.

Whatever its virtues -- and I shall return to this later -- close association with ordure is not without dangers. Foremost among these dangers is that of contracting a disease, especially a parasitic disease.

Visceral larva migrans is a disease of humans in which the larvae of dog or cat roundworms find their way into (from our point of view at least) the wrong host. If the little worms arrive in the central nervous system, or some other such crucial place -- and they occasionally do -- they can cause serious problems. *Toxoplasma gondii,* a tiny parasite apparently well-adapted to, and untroublesome in, the intestines of cats, may cause abortions, neonatal deaths, congenital deformities or respiratory, neurological or ocular (eye) disorders in other animals, including people. The usual route of infection is from a transiently-shedding kitten into animal feed and thence into the meat and finally into our own bodies. The young of the canine hookworms may penetrate the skin directly, where they are associated with a fate far worse than acne, *cutaneous larva migrans.* "Swimmers' itch" is felt after associating too closely with the parasite-filled droppings of ducks. *Diphylobothrium latum* is a tapeworm which, from dog dung, journeys through tiny crustaceans and lodges itself in freshwater fish. People who eat this fish and subsequently play host to the parasite may develop pernicious anemia as the tapeworm competes for the vitamin B?, in their intestines. Other dog tapeworms of the *Echinococcus* family may infect people and create tumour-like cysts in the intestines or brain.

Parasitic diseases are not the only curses to be visited on the careless manure handler. *Salmonella,* that bane of the turkey industry and mover of bowels, will make the jump from IT to you all too eagerly. According to Dr. W.R. Anderson, "If you feed your cat raw turkey, don't sleep with it." Despite all I've said above, I do not intend by this discussion to reinforce the public neurosis about excrement. If the stuff is handled at arm's length, and not at all by pregnant women, and if children are watched and washed with soap and warm water, there is no reason to flounder in Freudian paranoia.

Feces are produced as a by-product of eating and hence would appear to be an unavoidable part of the animal condition. Some animals have taken advantage of their natural functions, adding personalized scents which may be used to signify intolerance, dominance or territoriality. Elucidating the exact role of this scent marking is the work of certain behavioural zoologists and comparative anthropologists with peculiar research warps, and is beyond the scope of this brief scatological review. As a veterinarian, I am more familiar with its uses after it leaves the producer.

ITs most obvious use, in veterinary practice, is as a kind of barometer for what's going on inside the animal. It's what's left over after an animal (or person) becomes intimate with the environment, the dregs of love, if you will. But there are other uses. To the city dweller out for a drive in the fresh fall country air, the exuberant spraying of a honeywagon upwind may do something to dispel some of the myths surrounding country life. For the farmer, this spreading of manure on his fields serves the dual purpose of getting rid of waste and fertilizing next year's crop. Less visible to the casual driver, but as common as the manure spreader, is the use of dung from healthy animals, mixed with ample proportions of fresh, clean straw, to provide a warm and comfortable "manure pack" for the cattle to rest on. It certainly provides better footing and more comfort to the sick or labouring cow than a concrete floor, and I would not discourage it -- with the important provisos that the manure is from healthy animals and the straw is ample and clean. Good composting, with its attendant temperature rise, will even kill many harmful bacteria such as Salmonella.

Probably the most controversial use for manure is as food. With the high costs of many kinds of animal feeds, modern animal producers began to look to unusual places for help, and discovered that poultry manure in particular may be a suitable ingredient in cattle feed. Based on its nitrogen content (a fairly accurate measure if it is being fed to cattle), dried, caged layer manure may contain the equivalent of 27 per cent protein. Recent studies have suggested that it need not be put through the energy-consumptive process of drying, but can be fed in liquid form as a supplement to silage and/or grain feeding.

If feeding chicken manure to cows causes us to squirm a little, then coprophagy is entirely outside the bounds of polite thinking. The truth is that many rodents and rabbits literally couldn't live without it. In captive rabbits, soft feces called cecotroph are produced and swallowed whole at night, while hard waste is produced during the day. In wild rabbits, who do not have to perform cutely under the squeamish, authoritarian scrutiny of humans, this diurnal rhythm is reversed and the cecotroph is produced during the day. Microbes in the latter parts of rabbits' and rodents' intestines and in the cecum (an intestinal outpouching) help digest food which has managed to survive the first passage. These microbes, as well as the redigested food, serve as excellent sources of B vitamins, protein, fat and energy for these animals. Because of this similarity to the way a cow's digestive system works, rabbits have been called "pseudo-ruminants." Coprophagy in these species is not only an efficient food utilization mechanism, making rabbits some of the best food converters around, but is in fact necessary for their survival, helping to maintain their normal gut flora in a stable state.

Finally, I can think of no more clever nor universally applicable use for manure than that quoted in Theodor Rosebury's book *Life on Man*. A man who, I presume, wished to be cured of his infatuation for a certain lady, wore for an hour, shoes into which had been put her feces. The cure, it is said, was complete.

MAKING THE MOST OF THOSE FIRST FEW MOMENTS

Called at the witching hour to pull or cut a precious supercalf, implanted as an embryo, from its dispensable surrogate dam, my half-awake mind ponders the significance of this "business" called, by those who should know better, calf production. My soapy, slippery hand explores the vaginal opening, trying to read the Braille of two forelimbs and a head, or two hindlimbs and a tail. Pushing into the first available orifice, it is firmly bitten; a limb I grasp tugs back.

An egg and a sperm, fused under whatever circumstances, petri dish or Fallopian tube (the miracle being not in the surroundings, but in the event), have multiplied and diversified, flowering into blastocyst and neural tube, bones, heart, lungs, brain -- this gangly four-legged beast. And here am I, of no less humble, no less miraculous background, in the middle of the night, on my back in the wet, slippery straw, pulling at this calf's bony forelimbs, getting bitten: nature pulling nature's leg. In 20 minutes, exhausted, slimy, having survived the fleshy tunnels, the beautiful perils our fragile cells inherit, we are both here, now. They call this calf production? Some euphemism! It is pure epiphany, although I won't realize it until much later, when I've caught up on some sleep. The question now is, how do we keep us alive?

First off, if the calf isn't heaving a sigh of relief -- breathing, that is -- feel her heart. If that's going, hang her upside down and clean out the back of her throat. Give her a good rubdown. If that doesn't work, hold her mouth shut and blow into her nose. Sounds kinky but it's a gas -- the kind of gas she needs.

Aside from the failure to breathe, a lot of things can kill a newborn calf. Ask a microbiologist, and he'll give you a list of killers the length of your arm, most of them, not surprisingly, microbes. You get what you look for and, by gum, they're finding new ones every day, their number limited only by laboratory technology. And some would lead us to believe that every new microbe needs a new vaccine, which at least ensures good employment for vaccine companies, *ad infinitum.*

Opportunities for employment should perhaps not be sniffed at in hard times. Nature is not vicious, however, and most animalcules only cause problems under exceptional circumstances. From the point of view of preventive medicine, defining those circumstances is essential. The major improvements in human health have come about through the provision of clean water, good food and adequate housing. Modern clinical medicine is basically a driving home of drunks after the party. Thus it only seems fair and respectful, now, to share our human experience in water, food and housing with other animals: calves for, instance.

The single most important loving thing you can do for a calf, after it lands in clean, dry bedding, is to make sure that it drinks that first colostrum. In people, guinea pigs and rabbits, IgG antibodies, the persnickety Pac-Men of order in the blood, are able to cross the placenta, so that a baby is born with what is called "passive protection." (It also can result in prenatal Rh factor or other blood incompatibility problems.) A mother's colostrum and milk provide primarily IgA, which are antibodies that work outside the blood, in the gut and lungs. Breast-fed babies hence have a double dose of protection until they have convinced the microbiological world-at-large they are here to stay.

In our domestic farm animals, the prenatal placental invasion does not take place. Calves, pigs, foals, lambs and kids are born with no passive protection. Worse, they are born with what some of the more worldly wise among us might view as a naive openness. For the first 12 hours or so, a calf's gut will absorb, undigested, some pretty big molecules. What it wants is a massive dose of IgG, which the mother's colostrum provides. If instead, bacteria precede the colostrum, and/or colostrum feeding is unduly delayed, you can pretty well write that young-un off (unless you plan to raise it in one of those sterile air bags). This is true, as I said, for most of our farmyard friends. As a lecturer in equine medicine once intended to admonish us, instead slipping out a spoonerism and thereby expounding a philosophy of uncertain respectability: It is essential that the foal sucks. Carefully tonguing that twister so as to avoid advocating spiritual voyeurism, I would add that you should watch the foal after it sucks. If it turns yellow it may have a blood incompatibility with its mother, and should be given milk from a different mare.

The "more natural than thou" might think that allowing the calf to suck on its own is preferred. For lambs, kids and foals, leaving well enough alone is probably good practice. The newborns will usually find what they're looking for -- colostrum as well as motherly affection -- if left alone, which is not to be equated with not watched. Also, if you don't interfere with a mare's foal, she is less likely to interfere with your head. Piglets may need help getting to the teat, however, and calves may also pose special problems. A calf, when it first stands, does indeed search for that big sucker in the sky. It may search, naturally and unfortunately, around the highest part of the underbelly, where the goods are hung in most beef cows, and where they all had them a couple of hundred years ago, but which coincides with the armpits of sweet Daisy May. We've played around with Mother Nature and now we find that, like it or not, we've helped beget an instinctual misfit. So you may need to help that slippery bundle of bones to the teat. Forcefeed it if you have to (but only if you have to), by bottle, pail, or stomach tube. Get that colostrum in there, fresh from the mother if you can. Colostrum can be frozen and set aside for cases in which the mother is down with milk fever or comes in with a case of mastitis. If you freeze it in shallow pans, it will thaw more quickly when you need it. A Holstein calf should get at least two litres in the first 12 hours -- two good feedings during that time should do it. In general, if you feed eight to 10 per cent of the animal's body weight, you should be safe. There is no substitute.

While the mother cow cannot always be depended on to ensure her calf sucks, her presence when it does drink is beneficial. Calves that receive colostrum in the presence of the mother, even if they get it from a bottle, absorb more antibodies than calves that are removed to another pen to be fed. Nobody has figured out why, but the evidence is solid: Mamma's got something. In the literature, this something has been called a labile factor that is undescribed and unmeasured -- a sophisticated way of admitting that sometimes the more tightly you try to grasp nature in your fists, the more likely it is to slip through your fingers.

Picture then the calf, dry and warmly full of colostrum, snuggled next to its mother's peaceful bulk in the straw. Check your watch: three a.m. Go in and get some sleep. Touching as it is, this mother-calf tableau does not represent the complete picture of dairy calf rearing. As with marriage and birth in a human family, this is just the beginning of a long and very interesting journey. Most calves are suckled, not to mention conceived, at the all-intrusive bosom of humankind. Here they are fed, if not the milk of human kindness, at least an adequate replacer. With cows, as with so many of our domesticated animals, the lives of the people and the lives of the other animals have become interdependent to the extent that one may talk, in a very substantive way, about inter-species families. There are possibilities in this for a long-running television soap opera or a novel. That, however, I shall leave for another time, and another writer.

THE SCOURED CALF

The floppy floundering of a newborn calf in the straw, blurting out its first, slippery bawl, has always been an event of great significance for the dairy farmer. With the advent of superovulation and embryo transfer, not to mention the prospect of calf clones, the import of the event has taken on more complex dimensions, with new meanings layered over the old. But the miracle taken for granted is that there is a normal, four-legged beast there at all, and that has not changed.

The miracle we are after, however, is a perfect heifer. Sometime during the first three days after calving, the miracle of life and the cuteness of calfhood begin to take second place to real life and the rites of the milk goddess. During this time, when the colostrum in the udder is being displaced with milk, the calf is best removed to an individual pen or hutch. This is no time to ponder the mythic dimensions of a calf's lick. We may be fragile arms of the same biospheric beast, but one of us at least has to make a living at this business.

Calves kept in individual living quarters tend to fare better, both physically and behaviourally, than calves thrown into group pens. One study has even shown that individually reared calves may make better mothers than group-reared calves. Some things are best learned from the older generation -- even that of another species -- than from peers. (Farmers are better mothers.) No fancy nurseries are required, just clean, dry, cool quarters. A hutch, out of the wind and well bedded, is fine for the calf in even the coldest weather. Digging through four-foot drifts may tire even the hardiest of calf owners, however, and often compromise housing situations, such as hutch-like pens in an open-faced shed, are called for.

Of the various liquids available to feed a calf, fresh milk is the most obvious choice. If, however, you have uses or markets for the milk, you may want to feed the calf an alternative. A high-quality powdered milk replacer -- all-milk protein and 15 to 20 per cent fat content -- is acceptable, but sour colostrum is probably better. A modern dairy cow produces colostrum in amounts far greater than her calf can consume during its first three or four days. If the extra colostrum is poured into a large, clean plastic garbage pail, it will soon begin to ferment. You can either use a lactobacillus starter or just let it go. Colostrum is conveniently self-starting. This yogurt-like drink is diluted with warm water (two parts colostrum, one part water) just before feeding, and is given at the usual 8 to 10 per cent of body weight. Not only will calves grow well on sour colostrum, but since it has no real commercial value, your wallet will also appreciate this diet.

Feeding a little calf starter or grain (18 per cent crude protein is high enough) during the first week is also a good idea. Put a little in the bottom of the milk pail to get her started. This is increased to a maximum of four-and-a-half pounds per calf per day at six to eight weeks, when hay is usually offered and the calf is weaned. A newborn calf is essentially a simple-stomached animal in a class with pigs and people, and does not acquire its complex ruminant fermentation system capable of digesting hay until some time after its third week. An accelerated growing programme, using a 20 per cent crude protein feed and weaning the youngster onto hay at three weeks, works on experimental farms, as does once-a-day feeding. Accelerated growth, however, is sometimes a euphemism for accelerated fatness, which can result in later breeding and milking problems. Once-a-day feeding in the name of efficiency can also become an excuse for laziness or a rationalization for the inherent inefficiencies in the so-called economies of scale. It also affords one less opportunity per day for a nuzzling encounter with the real world. What works in hothouse experimental farms does not always work in the world most of us inhabit.

Every once in a while, nature -- in human form more often than not -- makes a mistake. The world, some of you may have noticed, is not always a fair place. Scours, perhaps the most common problem among young calves, is a type of diarrhoea that is aptly named and sometimes so severe that it seems an internal tap has been turned on full blast and is scouring the calf's insides.

The vandals at the scene of this intestinal crime are usually viruses or bacteria of some sort, such as some strains of *E. coli,* which can adhere to the lining of a calf's intestine where they secrete a hormone-like toxin. This masquerading toxin fools the body into secreting large volumes of fluid into the gut -- a situation that, if it continues, can lead to dehydration and death. Often the calf's handlers must take a large share of the blame. Lack of colostrum, dirty surroundings or coming through an auction mart, are all potential causes of scouring. Occasionally, of course, a bug so bad that it will drum the dance of death on the shiniest of sterile floors comes along. One or two strains of *E. coli* may be like that.

This is when vaccines may be useful. In most cases, however, I have seen no convincing evidence that the various scours vaccines on the market (and certainly none of those for pneumonia) could be recommended on any kind of routine basis for dairy calves. Usually, scours in dairy calves and the carpetbagging vaccine companies that thrive in its presence are a sign of management sins.

Given the fact that we all occasionally fail, and that bacterial or viral lightning can strike the most virtuous Jobs among us, how does one manage a scouring calf? Perhaps not surprisingly, as in human diarrhoea, antibiotics are generally of doubtful utility in the face of the waterfall. Given early enough, a couple of scour pills won't hurt, but the most important nursing care practice is to keep those fluids going in the one end at least as fast as they are flowing from the other. One version of "chicken soup" for calves includes a package of jam-and-jelly pectin, two teaspoons each of low sodium salt and baking soda and a can of beef consomme all mixed with a couple of litres of warm water. *Do not use table sugar*: it can make the scours worse. Keep the calf warm. If it is going downhill faster than you can keep up with it, have a vet administer fluids intravenously. It is all a big race to see if you can keep the body's bathtub full until nature puts the plug back in. No treatment is 100 per cent effective. Occasionally, a calf will pool fluid into its gut and die before it even has time to scour or the vet has a chance to demonstrate her wonderful skills. No miracle is complete without its nemesis.

The most important ingredient in calf rearing -- you can quote me to your friends -- is you. The right person, with care and attention, can successfully raise calves under the worst conditions. Care, experience and time, all items in short supply, are essential. Love your calves. They will lick your pants and suck your fingers. They may love the salty taste more than they love you, but with a bunch of healthy calves knocking at your crotch, a little anthropomorphism is forgivable.

THRUSH: THE CASE OF THE SINGING FEET

The ailments of a horse's foot: thrush, scratches, bruises, navicular degeneration, founder -- an endless list -- would be minor annoyance in other parts of the body, or in a different animal. But for the horse, the encroachment of pain and disease on the feet touches the foundations of a myth. It was, after all, in the cave of Cheiron the Centaur, half-man, half-horse, that Asclepius, bearer of the curative serpent (like the Judaic Moses) and god of the medical professions, learned his healing arts. We imagine ourselves to be the Greek Bellerophon, riding our Pegasus up into the sky. In the myth, it was only the rider who fell to his death on earth; in our present reality, the horse comes down with us and, more often than not, takes the brunt of the impact.

Standing in the cool muck, resting her soul after a bruising day walking on rocky ground or cement, the horse dozes. Unsuspecting victim. Aided by inadequately trimmed hoof walls, or shoes which protect the frog from proper, firm pressure, the primal ooze pushes its way up into the sulci (grooves) of the foot. Under cover of this terrestrial darkness, Mother Nature's microbial green berets attempt to recycle the living horse. We call it thrush, a degenerative condition of the frog, characterized by a black, odiferous discharge from the central and lateral sulci. We would agree with the appropriateness of one of the word's roots, a Dutch word meaning rotten wood. Or perhaps, hearing our hobbled Pegasus sing with pain, we are reminded of the robin, or some other kind of thrush.

From another point of view -- that of Nature Herself -- this "degeneration" is really a kind of reclamation project, recycling the myth back to its earthly origins. The Swedes have provided this viewpoint with its own appropriate linguistic root: torsk, for growth; this word-root leads quite naturally (and irrelevantly to this discussion) to another thrush, a disease of fungal overgrowth in the moist cavities of birds and people, often secondary to antibiotic treatments.

If this composting of the living foot is already underway when first discovered, all the dead tissue should be trimmed out with a hoof knife, and the hoof sprayed with, or packed with cotton soaked in, 50 : 50 phenol : iodine, tincture of iodine, 10% formalin (no higher concentrations please), 10-15% sodium sulfapyradine, or copper naphthenate. This latter chemical is available in many supply stores and vet clinics under various commercial names.

In sheep and cattle, similar disorders of the feet were named by someone with a definite bent for straight talk: foot rot. In horses, the disease is the work of an unidentified mixture of ingredients and is not, in the usual sense, contagious. Groups of horses are affected not by transmission from horse to horse, but by being exposed to a similar environment. In sheep and goats, two organisms acting in concert are thought to be the culprits, one of which (*F. necrophorum*) is a frequent barnyard layabout, and the other of which (*F. nodosus*) is, as they say, an outside agitator. *F. nodosus* thrives on attention: if you leave him alone, *sans animaux,* out at pasture, he'll disappear in a couple of weeks. While he's out there pining away, the sheep, in a kind of disciplined patriotic youth program, are having the rotten tissue trimmed out of their feet and are being run, weekly, through a 2 inch by 18 inch by 6 foot hoof bath filled with 5-10% formalin or concentrated copper sulfate (a pound of commercial blue stone in 5 gal. of water). Longitudinal corrugations in the bottom of the bath help spread the toes, and wood chips at the surface keep down the splash. In bad cases, you may need to inject some antibiotic into the tissue between the toes, where the infection begins.

Foot rot in cattle is similar to that in sheep in that it begins as an interdigital (between-the-toes) infection. Unlike the disease in sheep, however, bovine foot rot does not appear to be contagious, unless certain farms can be said to have epidemic quantities of stone, sharp gravel, tough stubble and primal muck. Trimming and cleaning the cow's foot, followed by antibiotics injected into the muscles, and local "dressings" are, as in the horse, the proverbial cat's meow.

All of our farmyard friends can only benefit from having their feet properly attended to. A horse's foot should be cleaned out with a hoof pick at the end of each day. The hoof walls should be trimmed periodically. Sheep, especially if they go out to shows, should be watched closely for lameness; spot check for foot problems whenever you can. At shearing, when the ewe is on her bum having her hair done, can be a good time. In all animals, look for bruises, cracks and abscesses as well as the black odiferous discharge of the rot brigade.

There is a kind of existential thrill that comes with being walloped into the gutter by a cow, a kind of euphoria in the exhaustion one feels trying to hold up the leg of a Belgian who has, during examination, developed a marked lean, and even a ticklish sort of *joie de vivre* from the sheep keds gathered during the examination of a ewe's feet. These are the sorts of in-body experiences that send a person reeling through Greek myths and Judaic history, in search for ultimate reasons. The lion who spared Androcles in the arena because the young human had pulled a thorn from his paw may find an unlikely parallel among farm livestock. Daily, we are seeing bankrupt farmers thrown to the beasts to entertain the patricians in the neo-conservative political gallery. How many of these might be saved by a magnanimous horse, grateful for good foot care? Most of us, no doubt, will simply have to be satisfied with firm-footed, long-lived service as our reward. Could be worse.

ECOLOGICAL AGRICULTURE

Looking back forty years or so to the beginnings of our current agricultural excesses, knowing what we now know about the earth, it would be easy to condemn people for having made a lot of wrong choices. But condemning our grandparents is too glib, and pointless besides; our grandchildren will no doubt condemn us for our short-sighted stupidity. Since our grandparents had no space-ship vision of Gaia to contemplate in their moral debates, and we do, our sins shall be deemed the greater. The fact is that, wishful thinking aside, people are short-sighted by nature, and the most we can expect from ourselves is to make the best decisions we can based on current knowledge -- knowing that our knowledge is always incomplete and that it is a sign of wisdom and strength to be able to change your mind when faced with new evidence or arguments.

I believe there was a time -- and I don't think I'm romanticizing this -- when we as a society had a coherent view of livestock rearing. Animals had their place in agri-culture, the culture of farming. If we no longer have such a coherent view, I think it is largely because of two things. In the first place, animal agriculture itself has become fractured into two basic camps, the centralized, urban consumer and money-driven agribusiness, with its related chemical industries, and the decentralized, increasingly marginalized, rural, farmer-driven agriculture. A recent issue of the magazine *The Ram's Horn: A Monthly Newsletter of Food System Analysis*, has a front page heading: "If you ask, who speaks for agriculture? You also have to ask, what "agriculture" do they speak for?"

In the second place, we as a culture have displaced millions of people from the countryside, where they were either on the farm or close to the farm, into the cities, where a whole generation is now growing up with no sense of the reality of livestock agriculture. Modern urban consumers -- and that, after all, is most of us -- have only images selected in the service of competing ideologies to go on. And, as with the three blind men and the elephant, we have different groups in society with opposing views of animal agriculture in the environment, each of them claiming to have the right and whole image.

Political and economic leaders have taken great pride in saying that some 3% of our population can now feed the other 97%, with enough surplus left over to service the national debt. The implication is that there have been too many farmers. This, quite frankly, is stupid. I don't think it's a good thing that only 3% of our people are working the land. I think it's a tragedy. I think we'd be much better off all around if that number were 30%.

I would ask, as Wendell Berry has, if we have too many lawyers, too many agricultural economists, too many agribusinessmen, too many university professors, or too many supermarket supervisors? Would it be seen to be a great accomplishment if we could get the same legal and economic advice with half as many economists and lawyers? Could we get twice as many courses and three times as much research out of half as many professors? Well, we'd have some turnover, but there are always young people coming up through the system. Isn't it wonderful to shop in a huge store where you can never find a clerk or a manager or anyone to help you find what you're looking for? If those who are currently lawyers and economists and agribusinessmen and professors could have the privilege of working, say, making parts for the computers and machines that have replaced them, or perhaps be on unemployment insurance, would that be seen to be a great accomplishment?

Saving some labour can certainly be good, freeing people up to produce many of the other things we need in this society, like CD players and video machines, but we have set the abolition of labour as a national goal, and hence have set unemployment as the ultimate accomplishment of our national economy. We have not seen the importance of labour as being the place where democratic economic institutions are energized and made real.

We have saved labour in the countryside for what? To provide a cheap working pool for urban industry, with about 10% left over to live on the dole, and at the same time we have aided and abetted the privately owned Stalinization of the agrifood industry. And we are surprised that the children of this displacement have a fractured, even bitter, view of agriculture? What's the big surprise? What we end up with is spokespeople for anti-farming groups who grew up on farms, and now, seeing what's happened, preach against farm intensification with thinly veiled bitterness, disillusionment and self-righteousness.

Animal agriculture is seen by some people as a place of disaster and a source of danger, sucking up the soil, spewing manure and chemicals into our drinking water and food, and heating up the globe. It is distressing to me, as someone who has some sympathy with this view, that some of the proponents of this view blame the farmers. I must say that this is where my sympathy ends. I don't like self-righteous, arrogant urban professionals telling farmers how bad they are any more than I like Monsanto telling us we need BST because we don't have enough milk, or have too many farmers or whatever, or than I like some self-serving integrated agrifood business telling me how safe our food supply is. I want to hear from farmers themselves, not some self-appointed umbrella groups that claim to speak for them.

A second view of animal agriculture is rooted in a romantic mythology carried around by the second and third generation of displaced refugees from the countryside.

This view sees animal agriculture as a moral activity. It's been around in various versions for a long time; in the last twenty years, magazines such as the *Mother Earth News,* the earlier versions of *Harrowsmith*, and *New Farm* magazine have worked this territory. But so, ironically, have various trade magazines in the cattle industry. This vision of animal agriculture not only sees animal farming as part of the natural way of things, but sees livestock rearers as independent business people. In many ways, the 1960s back-to-the-land hippies and the redneck cowboys were motivated by the same vision of life in the country, fresh air, clean water, hard work, simple pleasures.

Unfortunately, as Wendell Berry has pointed out, what is "natural" does not always come naturally. The millions of people who moved to the city in the last generation or two not only lost meaningful work and a coherent vision of agriculture, they lost the necessary skills to do agriculture. My first year out of vet school, I worked with young people from New Jersey and Munich who wanted to start a new life raising sheep on marginal land in the Peace River country of Alberta. The guy from Germany was there for economic freedom; the couple from New Jersey for ideological reasons. Their enterprises were disasters, no matter what the motivation. I tried to help them as best I could, but there was a sense of hopelessness about it.

Why do people still cling to this vision of the combination of being close to nature and economic freedom? I think there are two very different reasons. In the first place, there are those like Wendell Berry who see that a "right" way of farming is going, and that the countryside is going with it. They cling to this vision not because they think that this is the reality of farming, or the future of farming. They cling to this because they believe that this is how farming *should* be done. In this view, the good, independent farmers are under attack from what Brewster Kneen calls the *agrotoxin industry*, those urban based economic powers in whose best interest it is to keep farmers chemically dependent.

Secondly, and ironically, we see urban-based integrated agrifood enterprises promoting their food on TV based on this free and clean and independent vision. It is of course in the best economic interests of those who are making independent farmers a relic of the past, to have us believe that this is not happening. Centralized planning has rightly fallen into disrepute in the communist bloc, so it would not do to have it come alive and thrive right here under our noses. No, we must believe that the farmers who are leaving the land are doing so because they are economically inefficient and morally corrupt, the two being the same. If we thought that our consuming habits were helping to drive family farms out of business, we might get a squeal even out of urbanites. In this vision, those same good, independent farmers are under attack by irrational, fearful, organic, urban consumer vigilantes.

This second view of agriculture, then, sees it as essentially an environmentally friendly activity, if done right, but under duress from some outside forces.

A third view of animal agriculture and the environment is one espoused by many commodity and government-based farm organizations. Animal agriculture has come a long way from the subsistence farming of the 1930s; it is now a place of bounty where scientific miracles have taken place over the past generation, where we can now produce from one acre of land or one cow what once took a dozen. Through intensification, we have been able to enhance natural processes and free up marginal land for conservation without endangering the future. There are environmental problems, such as manure disposal and bacterial and chemical contaminants, but these are minor. Placed next to the obvious successes of the system, they are an irritation that can be worked out with a bit more application of sophisticated technology, vigorous regulation enforcement, and good extension work. We have the most productive farmers and the safest food supply in the world, this story goes; who can complain?

Consumers see agricultural fairs and full foodstores, and this "miraculous" vision, if I can call it that, sounds just about right.

Nevertheless, most people have difficulty reconciling this with newspaper stories of thousands of farmers going bankrupt and having big protest rallies, and with talk of increases in foodborne diseases or chemical contamination. Maybe, like the same business and political leaders are saying, those farmers just need to be more "efficient" -- that's why they're going out of business; they need BST; they need Cargill and Monsanto; they need computerized records. And yet, as more and more urban people are out of work, and small urban businesses go under, even urban consumers are beginning to think that maybe farmers aren't to blame for all their own misfortunes. Driving through the countryside, city people have the sense confirmed that agriculture looks good, but smells bad. Something is going on; but what? They become understandably anxious.

So we have at least three "mainstream" views of animal agriculture and the environment: it is bad for the environment, it should be good for the environment, and we don't know what it is or should be, but it's productive. All three of course have a grain of truth in them, which is why, heard in isolation or articulated by a good lawyer or preacher, they are all convincing in their own way.

I think we might make some headway if only the actual people that farm land be given the rights and privileges of farmers. No absentee landowners. I think that would help solve some of the environmental problems. It should be illegal of course to build industrial or housing developments on good farmland. Finally, I think farmers should have a guaranteed income based on the class of land and a composite measure of its health (productivity, quality and safety of the food coming out of it, energy and nitrogen efficiency, wildlife diversity, soil maintenance).

I think people in my profession and related professions should consider more carefully how to help farmers to farm better, more in keeping with the essential life cycles of the planet. I think this will lead us away from the "bigger is better" philosophy that we've had foisted on us in the last few decades. From the point of view of disease control and animal health, from the point of view of the quality of both individual and community rural life, from the point of view of caring for the earth, all the evidence I've seen seems to say that smaller, complex systems are usually better than bigger, simpler ones. We've gone the way of the Holsteins and Leghorns not because, ultimately, it's better for agriculture, or animal life, or for the humans that care for them, but because it's the easiest, slickest road to short-term profits. And intensive monoculture has been profitable because we've structured our economy in such a way that the major real costs of intensive animal production -- waste disposal, dislocation of human populations, environmental degradation, urban sprawl, Third World dependency, etc. -- are externalized and paid for by society at large, a kind of "hidden tax" on other people, including our own children.

I think we'll find that, if we pay attention to the land on the farms, as well as to the animals, as well as to the people, there will not be one way to do agriculture, heavily dependent on international oil markets and the maintenance of starving millions in Africa. Rather, there will be many ways, using many sources of energy. This, of course, puts into question all of our efforts to expand, internationally, semen and embryo transfer for farm animals, as well as intensive housing systems, large scale feedlots, the use of hormones and growth promotants, etc. The real problems in agriculture are no longer -- if they ever were -- related to production *per se*, but to sustainable, optimal production, a concept which must include social as well as ecological sustainability.

As I've said elsewhere (too often, some would say) I would also suggest that we re-integrate farm and urban life, with small scale farms, abattoirs and market gardens planned into suburban neighbourhoods. Such a decentralized system would promote safer, more energy efficient food production and distribution.

If some of these ideas sound "off-the-wall", it may simply be because we've been blinded by ideology to only think one way about producing and distributing our food. All this talk of "feeding the world" has had the ring of teenage bravado , "Hey Dad, look what I can do!" Who are we trying to impress? As the political walls are coming down in various parts of the world, it's high time we allowed ourselves to be sensibly creative about agriculture once more.

WHAT'S A SMALL ABATTOIR GOOD FOR?

The end result of livestock agriculture, as some animal rights activists are wont to remind us, is the production of meat. I have no intention, here, of entering into the quarrel between vegetarians and anti-vegetarians. They are both absolutely right. The path from the livestock farm to the dinner table leads through a problematic building called an abattoir. Many have discussed the problems we face in balancing a respect for animals with the practice of eating them (does the cat respect the mouse? I would say, most definitely). Others have elaborated on problems of keeping meat "clean" and "safe to eat" in what is clearly a non-surgical environment. Few have tackled an issue which is just as important as the first two: how the abattoir relates to economy and ecology in general.

The purpose of a slaughterhouse is to kill animals for human consumption; our usual measure of slaughterhouse success and the one which many agribusinesses would like us to use exclusively relates to how much meat the place produces in how much time. Matters of safety, quality and price are corollaries to this purpose. If businesses could produce large amounts of meat which is unsafe and charge high prices for something cheaply acquired, historical evidence is that many of them probably would. Consumers want not only a lot of meat coming out, cheaply, but we want it to be safe and good to eat. This is why government regulation is necessary.

The abattoir is also a place of employment, however, and hence a second purpose for a slaughterhouse is to provide meaningful and remunerative work for the people that work there. The remuneration is strongly connected to the first purpose, but the meaningfulness is a separate issue.

Finally, the abattoir is part of a socioeconomic web and hence influences both the nature of its inputs and the components in the food web after it.

In all of these things, the size of the abattoir has an important bearing. Small abattoirs are morally better than big abattoirs.

Small abattoirs are of course bad for some things. Cleanliness, for instance, might be raised as an issue. Small slaughterhouses are often a little more lax in terms of their enforcement of cleanliness rules than big ones, in part because of the kinds of individualists that run them. I think this can be blown out of proportion, however; there's a lot of dirt flying around in the big abattoirs too, where it has the possibility of contaminating a much larger proportion of our food supply.

Secondly, if all our meat were produced from small abattoirs, it would be more difficult to enforce general societal standards of quality and safety.

Finally, small abattoirs take more labour and initial investment per animal going through, and hence result in a more costly product.

None of these three points are important, I would argue, in any essential way. They certainly do not cancel out all the good things about small abattoirs.

Small abattoirs are good, in the first place, for reasons of food safety. In fact, if I were asked to undertake biological and chemical warfare against the citizens of this country, I'd build the biggest slaughterhouse I could and justify it based on the economics of scale and the invisible hand of the market. Politicians, who are apparently so naive as to be unable to make the fundamental, essential distinction between primary and secondary production, between food and shoes, are suckers for gobbledegook like that.

The incidence of diarrhoea and death from foodborne illnesses such as *salmonellosis, campylobacteriosis, listeriosis, toxigenic E. coli* have been increasing in the last few decades in Canada and the United States. Authorities on the subject such as Frank Bryan of the Centers for Disease Control in Atlanta have attributed much of this increase on a combination of intensive livestock rearing and large-scale slaughtering and processing.

Small abattoirs are safer because of the internal dynamics of slaughterhouses. A small slaughterhouse is inherently more capable of providing a safe meat supply than a large slaughterhouse. Whether or not the small abattoirs do so is less a function of their structural abilities to deliver the goods than of our neglect of them.

A large slaughterhouse provides the best possible surroundings for contamination of a large proportion of our food supply. One infected animal is a lot more dangerous -- can do a lot more damage in terms of infecting other carcasses -- in a big slaughterhouse than in a small slaughterhouse. Large slaughterhouses can of course overcome their inherent flaws through massive input of resources into facilities, chemicals, washes and irradiation.

Small abattoirs are safer because of the effects of the slaughterhouse on livestock rearing practices. A small slaughterhouse is ideally structured to respond dynamically to variations in throughput from small livestock rearing units, and hence, by its very nature, promotes smaller family farms over larger intensive units. Smaller groups of animals are less likely to induce stress in the individual animals, and there is less likely to be shedding of infectious disease organisms. Inherently, such livestock rearing units should be able to have both fewer infectious diseases and fewer of the problems with chemical residues than those which plague large intensive units. Again, the fact that many of them don't fit this ideal bill is that we've neglected them in our extension work to concentrate on the big producers.

A large slaughterhouse works most effectively when it has a large continuous input; hence it promotes large, intensive livestock rearing units and all the infectious disease and chemical residue problems that go along with that. Again, great expense and effort is put into trying to overcome the inherent flaws of the large slaughterhouse system and the kind of agriculture it subsidizes.

Small abattoirs are safer because of their effect on contamination during rearing and transport. By promoting smaller livestock rearing units, the small abattoir also promotes less intensive transportation of animals from farm to abattoir, and hence results in lower rates of stress-shedding and cross-contamination of bacteria.

By promoting large, intensive animal rearing units, a large slaughterhouse promotes high-intensity transportation for animals from the farm to the fattening place and hence to the abattoir.

Both by its internal dynamics and by its effects on livestock rearing practices, then, large slaughterhouses promote food poisoning on a massive scale, while small abattoirs are structurally more sound from a food safety standpoint. That is, if you were going to design an agriculture and food system around food safety, you would rear animals in small groups and slaughter them in small groups.

Secondly, small abattoirs are good because of their effects on rural communities. If I were asked to destabilize rural livestock rearing, put livestock farmers out of business, and deliver their enterprises into the hands of a centralized power (government or private), and provide cheap labour for urban industry, I'd build the biggest slaughterhouse I could and justify it on grounds of effi-ciency of safety inspection.

The purpose of work is to provide an opportunity for people to use and develop their skills together with others in the commu-nity in the common tasks of providing sustenance and material goods. Small abattoirs are good for the rural economy because of their effect on the structure of rural economic relationships. This relates to the mal-economy of scale.

A small slaughterhouse recognizes the true value of animals in the rural economy and ecology. It promotes economic independ-ence and responsibility in the rural community.

A large slaughterhouse promotes the economy of scale in a sector of society where this is inappropriate. It promotes the underselling of basic agricultural products and thus helps to drive farmers to rear animals under crowded conditions, to cut corners, and to remedy shortcomings with drugs. It forces many good farmers out of business. Those who stay in business are forced into feudal relationships, where Big Brother supplies feeds and chemi-cals in return, in perpetuity, for cheap labour and meat. Hence it promotes enslavement, the privately-owned centralization of the food industry, and ecological irresponsibility.

Small abattoirs are good for the rural economy because of their effect on working conditions and labour relationships. A small abattoir is structurally more set up to take care of its workers, keep them happy, because the manager doesn't have the "luxurious" anonymity that his/her counterpart in the big place has. It pro-motes social interaction, the basis of a democratic society. It doesn't always happen of course, but the nature of the small abattoir makes it more possible.

The value of work is not recognized in a large slaughterhouse. The quality of a workers' day is irrelevant to the management of a large slaughterhouse -- and it undercuts all attempts at promoting safe behaviour. It promotes adversarial behaviour.

Finally, small abattoirs are good because they are potentially places of essential learning -- higher education in its best sense. If I wanted to instill anti-agricultural biases and food-fear into urban consumers, delivering them into the hands of radical so-called animal rights activists and food-fad totalitarians, I'd build the big-gest slaughterhouse I could and prevent urban consumers free access to it.

Large slaughterhouses are built on the absurd premise that food -- livestock in particular -- is a commodity that should be treated like any other commodity. Consumers are thus surprised when they discover -- through bacterial and chemical food poisoning -- that their food is an essential biological link to the planetary biosphere. They would also be shocked at the carnage in a huge slaughterhouse. The best run ones are perhaps the most depressing, because they are so adept at fostering their illusions. But you don't have to be a vegetarian or a bleeding heart to be uncomfortable with large scale slaughterhouses. There is no respect in them, neither for the animals, nor for the workers.

The small abattoir, in offering at least the possibility of respect for life even as it takes it, could be used as a place to teach urban dwellers about our place on this planet, the nature of food, what it costs, where it comes from. Unless urban dwellers have a direct stake in agriculture, unless they know in a real physical sense where food comes from and how it ties us to the rest of life on this planet and to the environment, why our rural spaces are important, the farming community will find itself increasingly forced into enslavement to urban-based agrifood businesses.

Nothing about small abattoirs is inevitable, however. Without conscientious local inspectors and interested abattoir owners and workers, they can be disaster areas. And that, I would argue, is a tragedy.

The good things I have said about small abattoirs can best come about if the people who work there care about them. I think they are well worth caring for, if only to provide a humane alternative to the Big Guys, and I think that the people who work in the small plants should take pride in their work. There aren't many jobs left to us where this is possible.

LITTLE BO-PEEP MEETS DAVID SUZUKI:
A Word of Encouragement to Sheep Farmers

Little Bo-Peep, of Mother Goose nursery rhyme fame, cared deeply about her missing sheep. Her friends counselled her to "Let them alone, and they'll come home, and bring their tails behind them." Not satisfied with so lazy a solution to her problems, she set out, "determined for to find them." She was successful, we are informed, in her task, but "it made her heart bleed" that they had, in the process of wandering, lost their tails. In the end, however, all was well as she found the tails hung on a fence to dry, took them home, and tacked them back on to the appropriate "rump-o".

In much the same way, the Canadian scientist David Suzuki mourns the loss of our ecological innocence. As zoologist Vernon Thomas has pointed out, the environment is the "tail" in our society, wagging or drooping according to decisions made elsewhere, in politics or agriculture or industry. Some would say that we are even about to lose our tails -- and with our tails, our ability to be happy, even to survive. David Suzuki, in a book entitled *Inventing the Future,* has argued that we must set aside deeply held beliefs and values to reinvent a future, a path out of the wilderness of environmental degradation which, despite our best intentions, we seem to have created for ourselves. I would like to suggest that sheep and sheep farmers should be a vital part of that future and that, perhaps out of gratitude to Bo-Peep, or more likely simply *because*, sheep may now help us to save our own tails.

I recently attended a working conference on the Future of Public Health Education in Canada. When I returned, an acquaintance remarked that it sounded like a useless exercise, since experience has shown that those who predict the future are invariably wrong. That, however, entirely misses the point of planning for the future, a process we undertake whenever we buy a car, in which case we plan to have money, roads, and places to go, or when we walk to work, at the end of which exercise we hope there is something worthwhile to do, or if not, at least a paycheck, or even whenever we prepare a meal, for which we predict there will be a certain number of participants at a particular time. We are not always right, of course, even in such apparently simple activities. It's possible to buy a car and be unable to make the payments, or to lose one's job, that the barn or the office will have burned down last night, or that my teenaged son will bring a friend for supper and my wife will be working late, in which case I may need to adjust my preparations for supper. While we cannot predict the future, we do, collectively, by everything we do and say, create the future. What actually happens at supper is determined by what all the participants actually do. Acting on certain assumptions about the future is a necessary part of being alive, and, in so acting, we in some measure create self-fulfilling prophecies.

For a city-dweller like myself, there is something deeply satisfying about the thought of sheep. These are the animals you count before going to sleep. They bring to mind poems and pictures and songs of a pastoral way of life, green hillsides, a boy with a flute, and clouds like sheep drifting with the wind.

These images that enter our minds aren't about real sheep of course, but that's at least part of what I'm trying to tell you. It's not just the real sheep which matter, but how we think about them.

As a real sheep farmer, you might laugh at this image of your activities, but I would ask you not to scoff too quickly. Urban consumers -- who are in fact most consumers -- have only their images of rural life to go by. They have no first hand knowledge of it. And it is the images and the metaphors of sheep rearing, as well as the fantasy-titillated appetites of urban dwellers, that may well determine the fate of sheep and their caretakers in this country.

Sheep farmers today are walking a narrow, twisting mountain path between the valley of Disneyfication and the rocky wasteland of poultrification, between the fantasyland of Little Bo-Peep and the harsh environmental realities catalogued by David Suzuki.

Consumers want sheep to be cute and consumer-friendly, like Bambi, and they clamour for a product with the convenience and costs of Chicken-Licken. I am here today, somewhat sheepishly, as a lay person speaking to the experts, to urge you to stick to the middle path, to keep your variety and integrity. Do not let the gatekeepers for cute environmentalism pull the wool over your eyes, seducing you into the easy virtue and hard life of backyard farming. But, as well, don't let the industrialists ram the idea of mass-produced, quick easy bucks down your throat. Shepherding has given the world a rich and varied culture, biologically and socially and linguistically. The chicken farmers have in one generation not only given us a chicken in every pot, which is indeed a remarkable achievement, but they have in the process given up their freedoms and a rich biological heritage to a feudally-structured, centrally controlled industry. Do you really want that?

Leave them alone, advises the author of Little Bo-Peep, and the sheep will come home on their own, dragging their tails behind them, perhaps, like the fat-tailed sheep described by Herodotus in the fifth century BC, in little wagons. This is the ad hoc approach to the future of sheep farming. Sheep will naturally find their own home. But if we take this laissez-faire approach to the future, others will invent a future for us, and, like Little Bo-Peep, we may be disappointed at the results. Like the Biblical sheep lost in the mountains, we need a hook on the future, a good crook, if I might be allowed to mix my metaphors, to help us steal our way home. By hook or by crook, we need to find our own way.

Sheep and goats are believed to have evolved some 2.5 million years ago. Before the ice ages, they were said to be as large as oxen, which gives one pause, imagining such magnificent animals, and is perhaps a little terrifying, to think of a flock of such animals going into a panic stampede. Pioneers in the areas left by the retreating ice, they had, by the late Pleistocene, conquered Europe, Asia and reached North America. Some recent military leaders might take lessons in how this was done, quietly, without fanfare, one might even say meekly, but nonetheless very effectively.

M. L. Ryder has written a fascinating, encyclopedic tome entitled *Sheep and Man*. Despite a title which sounds much like the label for a nineteenth century romantic painting -- boy with dog, girl with peach, sheep with man, conjuring the image of a rather large sheep and a rather small man standing next to it -- the book is not romantically fuzzy, and in its wealth of details does not neglect the important roles of women and children in the saga of sheep. In this book, he traces domestication back to about 9000 BC in southwest Asia. He makes the claim that through domestication there has been a reduction in the size of the horns, lengthening of the tail, as well as a change from a coloured, hairy moulting coat to a white woolly fleece that grows continuously. Over the centuries, as Ryder has catalogued, literally thousands of strains of sheep adapted to local environmental and social conditions have evolved in many parts of the world, from Macedonia to Mesopotamia, from Barbados to the mountains of the Basques. Not only did sheep find their own way around the world, but in medieval times their skins served as a basis for waterproof maps for Genoan sailors, and hence made possible our own presence here, so far from our European ancestral homes.

The narrow, hairy muzzle with the cleft upper lip enables sheep to graze more closely and selectively than cattle, with their broad, naked, moist muzzles, and hence helps them to adapt to a more varied landscape.

Tip-toed and cloven-hoofed, and therefore adapted for climbing as well as for speed on open plains, most sheep have a strong flocking instinct, although that of course varies a lot depending on breed. Combined with docility, this has made them an ideal animal for nomads and semi-nomads, who still today guide their flocks through semi-arid landscapes where few other domestic animals could thrive.

Being ruminants, sheep can swallow food rapidly in the open and head for cover to regurgitate and masticate at their leisure. Their silent nasal belch is not only of survival value where keen-eared predators prowl, but may serve to endear them, as a valuable addition to anyone's dinner invitation list, to Miss Manners and Emily Post. Sheep always seem to be grazing -- up to 9 - 11 hours per day -- or ruminating -- another 8 - 10 hours, which has led at least one author (who apparently was poor at his sums) to suggest that, given the number of hours of grazing and the number required for rumination, they never sleep.

The shepherd-king David of ancient Israel suggested that it was the shepherd rather than the sheep who never slept, worrying about his flock and maybe, though he does not say so, about getting fleeced in the marketplace. His descendent Jesus, who had a great fondness for sheep, and often used them in his story-telling, thought of himself both as a shepherd, one who cared for each individual in the flock, as well as a lamb, an innocent sacrificial victim to forces beyond his control.

It is one thing to say that sheep are the ideal animals for nomads and the perfect sacrifice to the gods, who historically appear to have confused naivete and flocking instincts with innocence, but it is something else to suggest that sheep are an ideal animal for the twenty-first century. Yet I would argue that, in many ways, they are -- not perhaps ideal for industrialized agriculture, but an ideal ecological and, dare I say it? moral alternative.

They are, as ruminants go, small. Small, as the economist E.F. Schumacher proclaimed, is beautiful. It's something on a human scale, something you and I can handle. It's economically compatible with democracy. Sheep can produce milk, wool and excellent meat. They are therefore versatile and adaptable in both lifestyle and production. Versatility and adaptability are evolutionary and ecological virtues, in the face of climatic and environmental uncertainties, and our inability to predict what the future agricultural landscape might look like. They are certainly better suited to the coming dry-age that we see even now creeping into southern California than are the water-guzzling high-protein-gorging strains of cows we have so successfully created. Furthermore, their versatility and adaptability, and the great richness of biological material still available around the world, mean that we can imagine futures not available to the dairy farmers and the chicken farmers.

What sheep seem to lack, perhaps, is an adequate year-round sex drive, which some (some who don't really know, I might add) might suggest is very Canadian of them. Cultural history nevertheless abounds with yarns about the closeness of sheep and shepherds, and the origins of sexually transmitted diseases.

We may indeed decide that we want to breed for a new race of promiscuous or giant sheep. This is not a new dream. It is in fact a very ancient dream. An old rhyme about The Ram of Derby describes a beast with wool reaching to the sky, where the eagles nest in it, horns so tall that it would take a person from January to June to climb up and down. On his death, the blood washed out in a great flood and spun the water-wheels. Little boys used his eyeballs as footballs. When the rhyme was first composed, it was a good joke, of course, a ludicrous fantasy. In this day of gene-splicing and scientific "breakthroughs", when our dream ponies break through into living nightmares, this dream is more dangerously possible than ever before.

I would advise caution against pursuing this dream of a super-sheep too aggressively. Suppose we do breed a sheep that lambs well all year round, with multiple, fast-growing lambs. My questions are: what do these sheep need, in terms of water, energy and feed inputs, to accomplish this? What kind of management framework do they require? How widespread is this framework likely to be? What are its environmental and social consequences? These are the kinds of questions I never see asked by the animal breeders and geneticists. It's as if they think animals are reared in some kind of biological and social vacuum instead of in the real world. This new super-breed may be an important part of the homespun mosaic, but never let it take over the whole. A one-colour picture runs the risk of being terminally boring.

The great weakness and the great strength of sheep rearing is that sheep have, as sheep will, evolutionarily and historically, gone astray, each to their own way, each tuned to some specific topographical and social milieu. They are thus ecologically resilient, but economically vulnerable. Economic strength consists in masses of people, money, capital, land, or animals. This is sometimes referred to as the economics of scale. The big mistake we have made in some other branches of agriculture is to believe that all the animals need to be amassed in one big, vertically integrated, privately owned farm, and that they all need to be genetically and phenotypically the same -- the McDonald's syndrome, which is really nothing less than a capitalist version of Stalin's dream. From the point of view of both infectious disease epidemiology and environmental concerns, that's a sure recipe for disaster.

I would argue that it is very important for sheep farmers around the country to flock together, sounding the ram's horn at the walls of McChicken's Jericho. I would also argue that it is equally essential for the sheep industry to maintain a broad genetic and breed base, which I think may mean that sheep will need to be raised in relatively small groups, responsive to local conditions. It is important not to confuse mass marketing with mass production. The former is economic good sense; the latter is biological and social foolishness. It doesn't mean that one farmer can't raise a lot of sheep. It means that they probably shouldn't all be raised in one place, and that much reliable, skilled labour will be required. And when I say small, I also mean very sophisticated, and probably quite intense, requiring a deep knowledge both of sheep and of the landscape within which they are being reared.

There is no substitute for good husbandry, for watching your sheep, for knowing them well. I recently talked to a sheep farmer who told me he deliberately chose not to put automatic waterers into his newly-built sheep barn so that he would be forced to go out to the barn and turn on the water several times a day. That might sound crazy to our modernized ears, but to become excellent businesspeople at the expense of good husbandry and good biology was not, in his view, progress.

I think we can raise sheep, and market sheep, as being small-scale, and ecologically resilient. We can mass market a true variety of sheep meats, wools, manure-fertilizers, and even milk, as an alternative to that other alternative, goats' milk. I think that rearing and selling sheep like another kind of chicken, or pork, or feedlot beef, would be a mistake. If anything, one might look to the fish industry, where consumers buy not just fish, but trout, or salmon, or cod. Why couldn't they buy different kinds of sheep products, labelled as being from such-and-such a breed, not for differences in flavour, but for the pleasant thought of supporting ecological diversity? I think it might be an idea whose time has come. Throughout history, people have sacrificed a lot of sheep to various gods; it would be a shame to now sacrifice them to Henry Ford's production line.

I think that it's possible to increase efficiency of production without sacrificing, not only the peculiar biological and cultural strengths of sheep, but the democratic freedom of sheep farmers. Some might say I'm after the best of all worlds, some kind of golden fleece. But I'm not. I think what we should be after -- what I'm after -- is the best of this world. When we get to that last trumpet, that final ram's horn, I'd be quite pleased to be on the right-hand side of the throne, the side where the sheep are gathering. If we take care of, and care with, our sheep in this world, the other worlds will take care of themselves.

PART III:

GARLIC

THE HERBAL BIBLE

In the spring of 1981, a 73-year-old Edmonton widower began experiencing abdominal pain, general weakness, shortness of breath and fatigue. After admission to hospital, he was found to be suffering from lead poisoning. Public health investigators were unable to uncover any exposure to possible lead-containing drugs, home remedies, peeling paint, faulty plumbing or poorly glazed pottery. Nevertheless, two months after his initial treatment and return home, the man returned to the hospital for further treatments for lead poisoning. His illness continued despite therapy, and public health officials intensified their investigations. During this investigation, one of the man's relatives revealed that he had been using Chinese herbal medicines as laxatives. When confronted on the subject, the old gentleman admitted to using some little red pills, Koo So Pills, marketed by herbalists for curing "female complaints" but also, apparently, as a laxative. He had not mentioned these pills to the officials because, he thought, they were merely herbs and not drugs. These harmless little red "nondrug" pills were found to be coated with very high concentrations of lead.

"My attitude to herbal medicine," says Juliette de Bairacli Levy in her *Herbal Handbook for Farm and Stable,* "is almost worshipful."

I juxtapose the story and the quotation not to discredit Ms. de Bairacli Levy but to raise a serious question. My question is in response to a letter in which a reader queried me with regard to how much "faith" he should put in the "Bible-like" writings of that renowned herbalist. Indeed, in response to questions about herbal veterinary medicine in general and her books specifically, I would say that she is considerably more honest than some of my scientific colleagues, whose attitude toward the techniques of their trade is worshipful as well, but who would be loath to admit it. A great many "scientists" are wonderful technicians but know very little of science or of the philosophical foundations of the temple in which they worship.

A few years ago, the results of a field-trial testing a vaccine against calf diarrhoea were published in a reputable veterinary journal. The results showed clearly that when animals were properly and randomly assigned to treatment and control groups, the vaccine had no significant effect. The authors noted, however, that when an entire group of calves was treated with the vaccine, they had fewer disease problems than the preceding group, which was not so treated.   On this basis, they concluded that the vaccine was effective.   So many things change over time and from one group of animals to another, however, that to characterize that change by singling out one item, such as a particular vaccine, is clearly an act of faith.   As any farmer knows, some years are good and some are bad, even with no conscious changes in management.   Nevertheless, this act of faith was recorded in a scientific journal and hence entered the realm of "known facts".

The *Herbal Handbook,* in addressing the pitfalls of orthodox veterinary medicine, admonishes, "Farmers should insist on knowing the full nature of the drugs, vaccines and so forth, given to their animals. . ." I agree completely, but would add that this should apply to all treatments, orthodox and herbal.   Not all herbalists are as honest or as knowledgeable as Ms. de Bairacli Levy, nor are all veterinarians as benign as James Herriot.   Accept neither fuzzy goodwill nor arrogant professionalism as an adequate answer.

The practitioners of both orthodox veterinary medicine and traditional herbal medicine have a number of human flaws in common, the chief of these being a heavy reliance on personal anecdotes, or as medical scientists refer to them, case studies.   Not too long ago, my six-year-old son was playing outdoors and sustained a serious blow to the head.   Very quickly, the site of the blow, near his eye, showed every sign of becoming swollen and bruised -- a real shiner.   A neighbour of ours, who is from Mexico, immediately suggested, "Cut a potato.   Hold the cut surface against the bruised area." There being no serious orthodox alternatives, we followed her advice, and the shiner never developed.   In fact, in several instances since then involving both my son and my daughter, we have used the cut-potato compress to prevent and to treat swelling and bruising.   The technique has been invariably successful.   I could also praise the value of lettuce tea to quiet a colicky infant, but I already seem to be somewhat far afield from my intended topic.

The final word, however, is that these stories prove nothing, although they suggest a great deal.   Only a properly designed, statistically sound study could determine, with any semblance of objectivity, if the treatments are effective.   Until this is done, you have only my personal testimony to go on.   And how do you know that I am not like the medieval traveller, Sir John Mandeville, who described a tree bearing a huge melon-shaped fruit that he himself had tasted and within which, when he opened it, he discovered a lamb? The fruit, when ripe, would fall to the ground, the lamb's legs would protrude, and the lamb would eat all the grass within range.   The vegetable lamb story was finally exploded by the careful work of Carolus Linnaeus, in the 18th century.   Until then, many people believed it.   Since some of our stories of herbal cures come from Mandeville's contemporaries, I think we have a right to be sceptical.

On the other hand, medical scientists sometimes draw weighty conclusions about a disease after examining only a sampling of sick animals, which is really not much better than relying on Mandeville's data or on herbal guess whats.   You cannot talk intelligently about disease without talking about health.   I do not want to see just those animals that got sick.   I want to see those that didn't get sick.   I want to hear about the failures as well as the successes of various treatments.   I want to see the two sides added up and compared.   Without the presence of darkness, we can learn little of importance about light.

Besides religious fervour, orthodox medical practitioners and herbalists often share an incredible closed-mindedness.   Juliette de Bairacli Levy is considerably more open to seeing the baby in the bath water of modern medicine than are many of her colleagues, but even she has a tendency to scoff uncritically at the ways of modern science.   The detailed physiological, microbiological and epidemiological research carried out on animals in the past few decades has a great deal to say that is of importance if we are only willing to sort out the noise from the music.   Often, modern research supports and refines our understanding of holistic animal rearing -- the values of colostrum and mothering, for instance, or the fact that hay and grass, those old farm stand-bys, really are the best cattle feed.   I believe that every aspiring herbalist could benefit from reading a standard textbook of pharmacognosy, the study of drugs and where they come from.

On the other side, an editor of a food-engineering magazine recently scoffed at the "all natural" fad in food marketing.   The average potato-eating person, he pointed out, ate enough solanine (an ingredient in potatoes) annually to kill a horse, if given in a single dose.   He concluded that on the basis of pounds per capita of chemicals eaten, "natural" and "non-natural" diets were not significantly different.   His implied conclusion (I think) was that we shouldn't worry about our food at all.   Having washed the natural apple of truth -- that we need to be as vigilant about "natural" toxins as about manufactured ones -- he has drunk the wash water and declared the apple inedible: a clear case of fuzzy thinking in the service of a cause.

Tsutsugamushi disease, or scrub typhus, has been known about and described in the Far East for hundreds of years.   Early in this century, when scientists began to investigate it seriously, Japanese peasant farmers suggested that it was an infectious disease spread by a kind of harvest mite (a tiny insect).   Scientists turned up their noses and declared that the disease was due to a chemical toxin, thus setting back research on the subject for some years.   In the end, the farmers were proved right.   All of us think we are above such arrogant blindness, but the failings of the flesh, I have found, are the prerogative of no particular religion or station in life.

Herbalists and their scientific fellow human beings share another fault: the sincere faith that all disease is curable by their method, and that failure, or death, is the result of not following instructions properly, or lack of perseverance in treatment.   Disease or death, they are saying, is the result of the failure to comply with some religious (herbal, scientific) law, or the result of lack of faith.   All this may be so -- I for one cannot prove or disprove it -- but it strikes me as being singularly unkind to lay the burden of guilt on the patient (or farmer) without providing some avenue of salvation by grace.   Animals sometimes doggedly get better, or die for that matter, despite all we do to them, herbal or otherwise.

The Christian Bible is a collection of history, prophecy, law, personal anecdote, poetry, story and song.   It is a record of one people's struggles with God and the universe, and as such is full of archetypal imagery, heart-wrenching questioning, anger, ecstasy and eternal truths about the human condition.   In the personal search for truth, I have found it to be an excellent place to begin and to come back to again and again for nourishment.   But it was never intended to be a cookbook for answers (chapter so and so, verse thus and such says, therefore . . .); there is no quick and easy answer book for the Truth quiz.   In exactly the same way, there can never be an ultimate answer book in the search to be at home, and healthy, in the arms of Mother Nature.

A few common-sense aphorisms are as good criteria as any to guide our quest.   If you do no good, at least do no harm.   In a polluted world, there is no safe place.   Be vigilant.   Moderation in all things.   Often, the best treatment for a sick animal is loving personal care and attention. Everyone's truth is a partial truth. Leave well enough alone.

Words -- scientific, literary, religious or herbalist -- should never be held in higher esteem than the reality they describe. While science progresses through the accumulation of general truth, which can be hypothesized, particularized, refuted, supported and re-generalized, each of us leads these abstractions back into the blood and flesh and dung of our own lives. Ultimately, neither Juliette de Bairacli Levy's *Herbal Handbook* nor Goodman and Gilman's *Pharmacological Basis of Therapeutics* is an adequate substitute for the experience of Nature. Do it. You can always talk about it later, you should live so long.

WORM WARFARE

PART I

In the search for alternatives to several of the toxins used to treat intestinal parasites, some horse owners have suggested to me the possibility of using garlic, onions, and wormwood. Not being well-versed in the anti-parasitic uses of these particular plants, I undertook some research to determine the basis, if any, for such a treatment.

Whenever the opportunity presents itself, I like to call on higher authority, a second opinion if you will. In this instance, the prophet Jeremiah, well known for conveying bad news, comes to my aid:

> "And the Lord saith, because they have forsaken my law, which I set before them, and have not obeyed my voice, neither walked therein; But have walked after the imagination of their own heart, and after Baalim, which their fathers taught them: Therefore thus saith the Lord of hosts, the God of Israel; Behold I will feed them, even this people, with wormwood, and give them of the water of gall to drink." (Jeremiah 9: 13-15)

If it seems improbable that God would punish His wayward flock by giving them an herbal purgative for worms, we need only turn to *The Pharmacological Basis of Therapeutics* by Goodman and Gilman (1955 edition), for an explanation. *Santonin* is the active ingredient in wormwood, a common name for various species of *Artemisia* plants. When taken in low doses by people, it may disturb colour vision. Objects may at first appear blue and then, if they are bright, yellow. Hearing, smell and taste may be altered. As the dose is increased, headaches and vomiting lead on to abdominal pain, cold sweats, muscle tremors, and convulsions. One hopes that the worms are duly impressed.

If this were the whole story, one would be tempted to leave wormwood to the medieval woollen industry, which used it as a moth repellent, or to beekeepers, who can burn it to drive bees from their hives. But the santonin "trip" is not the whole story. Roman victors in chariot races were sometimes given a *draught* of wormwood for good health and long life. The herb has been used in soup to treat liver complaints, and as a tincture in rum to rub on fallen arches. Perhaps the most remarkable success story comes to us from the annals of medieval warfare. Benvenuto

Cellini, an artist fighting in the service of Pope Clement VII (Henry VIII's excommunicator), was seriously wounded in battle. When wormwood steeped in Greek wine was applied to his wound it healed immediately.

The trouble with this story (and with so many anecdotes from the history of herbaldom) is that we cannot be sure whether the cure was effected by the wine, or the herb, or a happy combination of a good year for Greek wine and the right stage of plant growth, or a miracle of good faith unrelated to wine or wormwood. It may be the greatest cure since onions and garlic, but until wormwood is tested -- which is improbable, given the state of research funding and the prejudices of the scientific establishment against everything they didn't think of first -- we have only fireside testimonials to base our decisions on.

Onions were counted among the gods of Egypt (I'm beginning to wonder what wasn't deified in Egypt) and Egyptian priests were said to deprive themselves of onions as an act of ascetic self-denial. This revered member of the lily family has been roasted, split, fried, mixed with cod liver oil and steeped in boiling water. It has been hung in doorways, applied to wounds, breathed in, sipped, quaffed and supped on. Among the many diseases which have (apparently) succumbed to its magic are tumours, cholera, calluses, burns, ulcers, urinary incontinence, rheumatism, severe headaches, athlete's foot, warts, asthma, baldness, bronchitis, nosebleeds and 'seminal weakness.' With this kind of curriculum vitae, it hardly seems fair to exclude intestinal worms. At the very least, onions may act as a bulk cathartic. On the other hand, a good bran mash would do this job as well, but bran mash has a more plebeian history, with no priests to recommend it. Onions, fed at two pounds per day for five days, can cause anaemia in people and in dogs. I've never seen this particular kind of anaemia described in horses. Probably no one has tried to feed a comparable poundage of onions to a horse.

The story of garlic is similar to that of onions, for it has been used for all manner of diseases from skin complaints and pneumonia to rheumatism and sexual infertility. For the treatment of equine worms, Juliette de Bairacli Levy in her *Herbal Handbook for Farm and Stable* suggests feeding garlic at the waxing of the moon, when the worms are stirring. By analogy, I suppose, its sexually stimulating properties should be at their most potent then as well.

How effective would wormwood, onions and garlic be for the treatment of worms in horses? I have no idea. I don't think anyone does. I do know however that worms are as much members of the animal kingdom as horses are, and that if you are out to kill one, you are unlikely to leave the other completely unscathed. No anthelmintic (dewormer), organic or not, is completely safe: that's part of the price we pay for living in an organically interrelated world.

An ideal anthelmintic should be specific for the target parasites, poorly absorbed from the intestine, and, like the ideal political program, free of side effects, with an effective dose much lower than its toxic dose; it should be economical, easy to administer, and not prone to encounter resistance from the target population. The ideal anthelmintic, like the ideal political program, will, no doubt, never be attained. Nevertheless an ideal provides some criteria for judging present inadequacies. Santonin, the active ingredient in wormwood, is well absorbed from the intestine, so that I suspect the toxic and therapeutic doses are not so far apart. Perhaps the onion and garlic act synergistically with the wormwood, so that a lower dose of the latter is effective, but this is mere conjecture. Most commercial equine anthelmintics attempt to disrupt enzyme systems that are specific to the worms, or to relax (paralyse) the worms enough so that the horse can expel them on its own. Many are poorly absorbed from the intestine. Sometimes a horse will develop colic after being dewormed, which may be due to the dewormer, a mass exodus of dying parasites crowding toward one small exit, or a combination of both.

In order to decrease chances of toxicity, some horse owners might be tempted to use lower than recommended doses. This is a mistake, whether using organic or synthetic drugs, since a lowered dose will not be enough to affect the worms, but may be enough to let them acquire a taste for the drug, and thus become resistant to it. A horse owner with a sadistic bent might consider hooking the worms on the drug, and then cutting off their supply, letting them die of withdrawal symptoms. I recall as a child hearing the following cure for a tapeworm: Every day for a week eat one boiled egg and one piece of salami. On the eighth, day, skip the egg. The tapeworm, so the story goes, crawls up into your mouth to call, "Hey, where's my egg?". If you're fast enough, you can grab him by the neck and pull him out. I've never seen it tried in horses.

If you want a hot tip for organic romance, I can suggest an onion quiche, liberally dosed with garlic, and a bottle of good Greek wine at the waxing of the moon.   The same tactics may lead your horse to love you more, but a clean stall, good feed, careful attention to grooming and, yes, even a regular dose of chemical dewormer will probably do more to control her parasites.

PART II

The great strength of the holistic, organic world view is not in the cures it effects, but in the sickness it may prevent.   I have no doubt that many traditional herbal remedies can, under the right circumstances, be as effective as some of our modern wonder drugs.   Far more important to my way of thinking are the clean air, pure water and uncluttered lifestyle which are the holistic ideal and which, if implemented, could make many of our potent remedies unnecessary.

There is a wide variety of parasites willing to set up house-keeping in a horse's internal organs.   Probably the most serious among these are the three *Strongyle* musketeers, *S. equinus, S. edentatus* and *S.vulgaris.*   As with parasitic worms in most animals, the adults living in the intestines know who's buttering their toast and usually cause minimal trouble.   Like respectable middle-class vampires, they quietly suck blood, copulate and lay eggs.   The eggs pass out in the faeces, hatch, go through a couple of moults, and then, if they are lucky and you are not, the horse ingests them.   Then the trouble starts.

Strongyle larvae have wanderlust.   *Equinus* wanders around in the liver and pancreas before settling down in the cecum. *Edentatus* goes to the liver, but has been known to find the testes, losing its way, like so many mortals do, in the sexual laby-rinth.   *Vulgaris* larvae inflict the most serious damage.   They mi-grate along the walls of the arteries supplying the intestines, head-ing for the mighty blood river in the back, the aorta.   Although most never make it that far, it may take them half a year before they come floating home again.   Along this journey, they may cause blood clots (thrombi) which block off minor vessels supplying blood to the gut, or they themselves, after shooting the rapids, may become wedged, like Winnie the Pooh, in a place of great tightness.   These thrombi, whether composed of blood or larvae or both, can cut off the blood supply to various parts of the horse's intestines.   Depending on how much of the blood supply is cut off, and how quickly collateral supply lines can be opened up, the horse may suffer anything from a minor bout of colic to painful, spasmodic death.

Another kind of equine parasite, less serious than *Strongylus vulgaris* but more often noticed by owners, is the pinworm, *Oxyuris equi.* The adult pinworms live in the colon where the males, after some kind of orgasmic depletion of the vital force, die soon after copulation. The widowed females then wander out the rectum, where they lay their eggs in a sticky fluid. The fluid dries, the eggs fall off into the environment, the horse eats them, et cetera. The chief complaint of a horse with pinworms is an itchy butt; the chief complaint of such a horse's owner is the disfigured tailhead that results from tail-rubbing.

A third main type of equine parasite is the bot. Botflies *(Gasterophilus)* lay eggs around the head, neck and limbs of the horse. The eggs near the head may hatch directly and the larvae wander into the mouth; those that are around the limbs are picked up and stimulated to hatch when the horse licks them. The bot larvae wander down to the stomach, where they spend a snug winter. It may be nine or 10 months before they see the light of day again, pupate and emerge as a new generation of flies. Much of the damage caused by bots is mechanical in nature -- that is, a large number of them may cause stomach irritation and bowel obstruction. Adult flies may "spook" the horse, perhaps to the point where the horse injures itself -- a well-known political tactic used not only by *Gasterophilus* flies, but by the Americans in Chile and the Soviets in Poland.

No anthelmintic (dewormer) is completely effective, even if given regularly. Most are relatively safe; none entirely so. The best treatment is prevention, and this is where the "whole earth persuasion," as a colleague of mine identifies my bias, comes into its own.

Clean air. Lots of room. Good food. A diet that includes good quality hay and grain -- mostly oats if the horse isn't working, some barley or corn if she is -- can help her ward off the worst effects of an infestation. Horses should be kept in clean quarters. Soiled bedding should be removed regularly, and the feeding area cleaned with a disposable cloth and hot water. Don't keep leaky water bowls or buckets. Never put feed on the floor. Brush and groom the horse as often as possible, to dislodge any eggs stuck to her coat. At least one herbal article I've seen suggests applying used motor oil from a garage to kill the bot eggs, adding that this is "harmless." I've seen crude oil poisoning: It is *not* harmless.

If possible, different pastures should be used from year to year. Young horses especially should be put on clean pastures -- those not grazed by other horses during the same year. Horse pastures should not be fertilized with horse manure. Horses that haven't been recently dewormed or certified clean should not be allowed on the premises. If you are following your organic nose and practising good horse sense, and you want to know whether it's working, take a fresh stool sample into a veterinary clinic and have it checked for worm eggs. Do this regularly.

At the end of the day, your horse may still have some worms. You may not have been diligent enough. You may have had bad luck. You may have sinned. You may decide to live with your sins. (An otherwise healthy horse can live with some parasitic freeloaders.) You may decide to accept God's punishment of worm-wood and the gallwater of horse dewormers -- four or six times a year. You may decide, like the Romans, that the stuff isn't so bad after all. You do your best, and rationalize the rest. All our medical and herbal tricks are only delaying tactics: the worms always get us, and our horses, in the end.

SELENIUM: A POISONOUS NECESSITY

Nowhere in veterinary medicine is the delicate balance between living organisms and the environment more evident, nowhere is the generalized bacteriological model of disease more undermined, than in the relationship between animal health and some of the trace elements. They are necessary for life -- and they can kill.

Selenium, for instance, parked next to arsenic in the table of atomic weights, is essential to the well-being of animal life. One might think of it as a kind of elemental analog to a vitamin. Yet in some ways, an equally appropriate analogy to this element is another natural substance, strychnine. It has been said of strychnine that a lot will kill you, but a little bit is good for you. This is the rationale for including *Nux vomica,* strychnine's natural mother, in many so-called "rumenotorics" (rumen stimulants) for cattle.

It has been known for many years that selenium in moderate doses is toxic to all kinds of animals. Only in the last couple of decades have scientists discovered that this same element in minute doses is essential for life. Selenium, working in concert with vitamin E (alpha-tocopherol), acts to protect cell membranes in the body from destruction by naturally occurring toxins such as peroxides. Vitamin E in this role is called an anti-oxidant. Selenium is found within an enzyme called *glutathione peroxidase* which is sometimes measured in the blood to give an indication of the selenium levels in an animal. One can also measure selenium levels in hair or wool, which are probably more stable long-term indicators of body status.

Since vitamin E and selenium have similar jobs in the body, they can, to a certain extent, cover for each other. Nevertheless there is a critical level of each of these which is essential for normal body functioning. Below these levels, we begin to encounter outright destruction of cells within the body. In kids and pigs, heart muscle is often the first to go. These animals are dead before their owners know they are sick. In calves and lambs, the diaphragm and the leg muscles may be involved; hence the name "stiff lamb disease." Animals with this form of the disease may be unable to stand, but otherwise seem all right. White muscle disease, the common name for this ailment, derives its name from the appearance of the destroyed muscle tissue: pale, hard, fish-like. Often, especially if the heart is involved, blood vessels in the area rupture and hemorrhages are seen. In chickens, vitamin E and selenium deficiencies have been linked to "crazy chick disease" (no, this is not a sexist throwback to 1950s California), leakage from small blood vessels, muscular dystrophy and poor hatchability of eggs. There is no doubt that selenium and vitamin E are important.

At present, considerable debate revolves around what happens to animals who are only marginally deficient in selenium. Among problems being discussed as possible candidates are scouring (diarrhoea), infertility and general poor thrift in calves and lambs. The evidence for all this is largely circumstantial -- researchers speak of selenium responsive diseases -- and convincing only because of the number of testimonials rather than the quality of the evidence.

Animals derive their selenium from the food they eat. If their diet contains no selenium, they quite rapidly deteriorate into a state of selenium deficiency. The selenium content in the tissues of ruminants (sheep, goats, cattle) appears to approach equilibrium with any corrective dietary regime in 10 to 30 days. The plants in the diet derive their selenium from the soil in which they were grown. Whether or not a particular crop takes up sufficient selenium depends on the concentration of selenium in the soil, and the chemical form of that selenium. Various parts of the world have been mapped according to the selenium content of the soil and one can, with some degree of certainty, predict which general areas will experience selenium deficiency disease in their livestock. When it comes to predicting which farms, however, or even which animals may come down with white muscle disease, the odds of being right dwindle and may be comparable to winning a lottery, electing a sensible head of state or being struck by lightning.

The fact is that soil type and composition vary not only between areas, but also between farms and within farms. As well, many farmers buy feed, so that it is now possible to import one's problems from half a world away. The value of growing your own is that at least you know, or can find out, exactly what you are feeding your livestock. Dietary factors other than selenium which influence the development of white muscle disease include high levels of unsaturated fats, low intake of sulphur-containing amino acids and low levels of vitamin E. Sudden exercise or other stresses such as deworming may precipitate the disease in deficient animals. To make matters worse, the biggest, fastest-growing, healthiest-looking animal are usually the first hit.

At this point you could become paranoid, refuse to buy or sell feed, lock up your goats, not deworm them and listen to their hearts daily with a stethoscope. On second thought, you could sell them and move back to the city. No such drastic action is necessary.

First of all, if you have been growing your own feed for a number of years and have not encountered any problems, you are unlikely to encounter them now. If you think you may have problems, start at square one: make *absolutely sure* the diagnosis is right. This may involve a two-pronged plan of attack.

If you have animals that are suspected to be afflicted with white muscle disease, arrange with your veterinarian to have a complete blood work-up done, not only a white cell count to help rule out infections, but also enzyme determinations. Glutathione peroxidase, as I mentioned, is useful, but I'd also look at selenium in whole blood or in hair. If any of your four-legged friends should die, get a complete autopsy done. Just because one of your animals died from white muscle disease does not mean that any subsequent deaths or illnesses are from white muscle disease.

Second, if necessary, have your feed analysed for selenium. An adequate level of selenium in whole feed is considered to be 0.1 parts per million (ppm).

If the diagnosis is white muscle disease, the usual and most reliable treatment (for goats) is to inject does with five mg selenium with vitamin E (commercial preparations almost always contain both) at four to six weeks prior to kidding. Inject all kids at two to four weeks of age with a similar dose. Provided that the diagnosis is right, and the farmer is diligent in his or her injections, this should clear up the problem. Selenium may, on the order of a veterinarian, be added to the salt. However, milk from goats eating this salt is not to be used for human consumption. Selenium at certain levels may be protective against some forms of cancer but at other levels will certainly cause some forms of cancer. Also, if the selenium is in the salt, one cannot be sure that some of the goats don't overindulge while others fast.

If you are doing all these things and are still having apparent white muscle disease problems, start again. Have the diagnosis rechecked. Selenium overdose is among the several diseases that can mimic selenium deficiency.   I once worked with a pig farmer who started with pigs dying from selenium deficiency; we tried to fix the problem by adding incremental doses of selenium to the feed.   Somewhere along the way, we passed the balance point, and a year later he was losing pigs from selenium toxicity.

The moral to be extracted from these natural observations is one my father often repeated: moderation in all things.   It's not bad advice for all our eating habits, whether for selenium, or fats, fibres, meats, vegetables and all the other food ideologies to which we are subjected.

THE SMILING FOX DOES NOT WORK FOR GREENPEACE

If there is one thing that we can learn from the feared disease rabies, it's that when Nature is being friendly to you, you should be suspicious. This is not natural.

Rabies is a disease that has terrified people since antiquity. One of my colleagues calls it a "psycho-zoonosis", by which he means a disease people contract from other animals whose psychological impact far exceeds the probability of contracting it. Given its invariably fatal course, however, I can perfectly understand a certain apprehension which might accompany the thought of getting it.

"The only remedy", said the Roman physician Celcus of rabies, "is to throw the patient unexpectedly into a pond, and if he has not a knowledge of swimming allow him to sink, in order that he may drink, and to raise and again depress him, so that, though unwillingly, he may be satisfied with water; for thus at the same time both the thirst and the dread of water is removed."

Historically, other treatments for this disease have included eating a cock's brain, the rabid dog's head, or the raw liver from a drowned puppy of the same sex as the offending canine. Modern treatments for rabies, once the clinical signs have set in, are slightly more sophisticated, but not a great deal more effective.

Rabies (the name comes via the Latin from an old Sanskrit word meaning "to do violence") can infect cows, horses, dogs, cats, monkeys, people . . . the list of possible victims is open-ended. Even birds, once thought exempt from rabies' natural cycle, have come under suspicion as carriers. One story, probably apocryphal, tells of a man in Mexico who developed rabies after being attacked by a rooster. Skunks are notorious. Some early American settlers, noting the close association between the little creatures and the dreaded hydrophobia, dubbed it the Hydrophobia-cat, or Phobycat for short.

Nor are those safe, who, like Woody Allen are "at two" with Nature and hence avoid contact with animals altogether. Recently a woman in the United States contracted rabies after receiving a corneal transplant from a man who died of what was diagnosed as a rare neurological disorder.

The case of the corneal transplant is not, as some might think, just another gun in the arsenal of antitechnocracy. The donor had no history of being bitten and, under the best of circumstances, rabies is not an easy disease to diagnose. Affected cattle may go off feed and water, bawl, yawn, strain as if constipated, and with a determined but wobbly charge, send the veterinarian leaping over a fence. Or they may quit eating, lie down and not get up again.

A few years ago, in a large veterinary hospital, one of the veterinarians was examining a dog with alleged digestive problems. Gazing intently at the dog's tonsils, he realized with a chill that the dog was unable to swallow: it was rabies. One sheep farmer recently told me of how he had entered his house to find his normally docile housecat rushing madly at one family member after another, claws and teeth at the ready. At other times, a rabid cat will simply disappear into a dark cranny somewhere and not be seen again.

Rabies may be confused with epilepsy, canine distemper, lead, mercury or arsenic poisoning, a bone in the throat or other digestive or nervous disorders. Since not everyone who is bitten by a rabid animal comes down with rabies, it has been suggested that the strain of rabies seen in Canadian wildlife resembles the African *ouloufato* strain in its low degree of virulence (ability to cause disease) for man, but this has not been demonstrated to be true. Who is going to play the guinea pig? More likely, the better survival rate after exposure is due to proper wound care and post-exposure vaccination with five doses of a human diploid vaccine.

Rabies is caused by a bullet-shaped virus which travels up the nerves from a bite wound, or from any open wound contaminated with infected saliva. The disease is seen in three stages, or forms, one or all of which may be seen in any one animal. The "prodromal" stage manifests itself in fever, restlessness, refusal of food and frightened or odd behaviour such as snapping at imaginary moving objects. The "furious" animal wanders aimlessly, howls, picks fights and bites indigestible objects. The final stage is the "dumb" stage: an animal seeks seclusion, looks apathetic, mouth hanging open, drooling. The increasing irritability of the affected animal and its inability to eat or drink are related to the activities of the virus in the brain and paralysis of the muscles in the throat region. Most animals die within three to eight days after the symptoms are noticed. Unfortunately, infection might have taken place weeks or even many months before behavioral changes are seen, and the virus can be shed in the saliva up to three days before the animal appears out of sorts. A "helpful" person in London, Ontario, brought a normal, friendly stray dog into a nursing home for the residents to play with. The dog turned out to have rabies -- which is not an argument against bringing dogs into nursing homes to cheer people up, any more than AIDS is a general argument against sex. It means that a few simple precautions should be taken when you're dealing with animals you don't know.

In Canada, skunks, foxes, bats and sometimes raccoons are the most common wildlife carriers. In Europe, a wave of rabies came with the foxes from the East after World War Two. In the United States, an epidemic of raccoon rabies has been spreading up the Eastern seaboard. Ontario annually reports more cases of rabies than any other geographic area in North America. It is no accident, then, that researchers from Ontario, along with scientists from Europe, have been at the forefront in developing computer simulation models of the population dynamics of rabies in foxes. An oral vaccine, dropped from airplanes in "specially marked" packages of meatballs, has been successfully used to eradicate rabies from some valleys in Switzerland and is being "marketed" to the foxes in Ontario. In fact, the label on the package, based on the reasonable premise that foxes cannot read and people can, says, "Rabies Vaccine, DO NOT EAT". Furthermore, the meat contains residues of the antibiotic tetracycline well above the human-food legal limit, not to help settle the foxes' stomachs, but in order to mark their teeth. Teeth from fox carcasses brought in by hunters and trappers can then be checked for tetracycline staining to see how many animals have taken up the vaccine. Similar work on skunks is still in its infancy. What this work has revealed, as much as anything else, is how ignorant we are even about the wildlife who most closely live with us -- skunks, foxes, raccoons.

Not all jurisdictions have taken as gentle an approach as Ontario and Switzerland. The Province of Alberta declared war on rabies in 1953 in a programme that left an estimated 50,000 foxes, 35,000 coyotes, 4,200 wolves, 7,500 lynxes, 1,850 bears, 500 skunks and 64 cougars dead after a one and a half year onslaught. Finally, perhaps war-weary, or suspecting that the real source of the problem was in that hotbed of socialism, Saskatchewan, Alberta settled for an eighteen mile wide buffer zone along the Saskatchewan border to trap and kill any skunks crossing the provincial boundaries. There is some irony, then, in the fact that Canada's last human case of rabies was a young man bitten by a bat in a lumber camp in northern Alberta. But then, he did die in British Columbia, so perhaps that means the Alberta program was a success after all. Several studies have suggested that if a slaughter policy were carried out in a place like Ontario, one could expect an increase in rabies as a wave of feisty foxy adolescents swarmed into the post-war vacuum.

On the individual farm or rural property, vaccination and vigilance are the cornerstones of rabies prevention. Nature that has not learned to avoid contact with people is Nature that has not learned its lessons very well. A wild animal that does not avoid people is sick; picking up a "tame" fox, skunk or raccoon to keep as a pet is the worst sort of foolhardiness. Wild animals have a natural right to live and die in the wild. Homesteaders who respect this right may themselves have the privilege of a longer, happier life.

Of all the barnyard animals, the dog is the most likely to snuffle brashly into contact with wildlife, and should be vaccinated annually. Cats tend either not to pick fights as much, or, if they do, go away quietly to die rather than taking their owners with them. On the other hand, there are exceptionally Rambo-ish cats that will attempt to sink a whole household before they go, perhaps in revenge for a lifetime of being deprived of catnip. Other farm animals can also be vaccinated, although this is usually done only in problem areas.

Immediate treatment of bite wounds from a rabid animal includes thorough irrigation (washing) with a detergent solution for 30 minutes, followed by a good rinse and a disinfectant. If the wound is bleeding, it should be left to bleed, uncovered. The offending animal needs to be identified in some way; if it isn't shot (not in the head, as that's needed for positive diagnosis), or locked up in a shed, one should at least make a note of the direction in which it wandered off. Call a doctor. They are good for some things. The post-exposure treatment is not as bad as it used to be, and certainly less traumatic than being held under water until you're cured.

THE DISTEMPER OF OUR TIMES

"Distemper" comes from the medieval Latin *distemperare* and meant, at one time, "a disproportionate mixture of parts; want of a due temper of ingredients" (OED). In those days, it was a label to hang on just about any kind of disorder, from the political to the meteorological and the physiological. Today it has settled and stuck with three very different and distinct diseases: horse (equine) distemper, dog (canine) distemper and cat (feline) distemper. These diseases are interesting in their own right, but they may be equally important for what they tell us about disease in general, and our attitudes toward it.

Distemper in horses is a bacterial disease caused by *Streptococcus equi*. Horses affected run a fever, cough, have pus draining from the nose and, most characteristically, have swollen lymph nodes ("glands") just below the back of the jaw. It is popularly known as "strangles", although the lymph nodes rarely enlarge sufficiently to choke a horse, and most horses do recover from the disease. After World War II, prevailing attitudes being what they were (war-like), owners and veterinarians treated the disease by taking penicillin from their weapons cache and giving the sick horse a "shot." More recently, it was found that, far from routing the disease, mistimed shots of penicillin caused the *streptococci* to either lay low until the barrage was over and then simply take up where they left off, or, worse still, to retreat into the bowels and organs of the horse where they conducted disruptive guerrilla actions. This form of the disease was called bastard strangles.

If this war-like attack is to succeed at all, it must consist of a barrage of high doses of penicillin started before the lymph nodes swell -- before most people even notice the horse is sick -- and should be continued for at least two weeks. The alternative to this napalming is simply good nursing care: fresh air, clean water, good food, a quiet place where the horse can be alone, and hot packing of the swollen nodes until they rupture. Then penicillin can be given. Not surprisingly, it appears that nature cooperates more often if we work with her.

Canine distemper is a viral disease of dogs, wolves, foxes, coyotes, mink and a number of other animals, characterized by high fever, discharge from the eyes and nose, sometimes degenerating into pneumonia and occasionally seen as a nervous system disease which can be confused with rabies.   The virus which initiates this disease resembles the human measles virus, which can be used to vaccinate pups against distemper.   More animals get infected with the virus than come down with the disease, and not all dogs that get the disease die, although case fatality figures have been pegged as high as 50 per cent.   Good nursing care (fresh air, clean water, et cetera) has been claimed to have curative power by some, and damned as a frustrating exercise by others.   Annual vaccination usually protects a dog from the disease.

Feline distemper is caused by a virus that attacks rapidly dividing cells in the cat's body.   White blood cells are especially vulnerable, and hence the scientific name panleukopenia (deficiency of all white blood cell types).   Cells lining the normal intestine are constantly being rubbed away and replaced; in feline distemper this replacement does not occur and diarrhoea results.   Brain cells are still dividing in fetuses and young kittens; these too fall prey to the virus, with various distressing results.   Kittens often die from distemper, but adult cats are more resistant.   Again, vaccination is available, and recommended.

A number of years ago, some researchers studied the course of canine distemper in germ-free (gnotobiotic) dogs.   They found that the dogs did not come down with the expected high fever and pneumonia-like syndrome usually seen in the "wild."   What they did notice was a drop in the white blood cell count:: the cells which are responsible for detecting and fighting off "foreigners" in the body.   This is similar to what we see in feline distemper.   Quite often, it may not be the virus at all which produces the clinical signs -- or even death -- but what are called opportunistic invaders: normally benign bystanders just waiting around for something to do.

Canine and feline distemper are not alone in this regard.   In swine dysentery for instance, the normal intestinal flora are believed necessary for the culprit spirochete to do its work.   Disease may thus come as a result of various bacterial and fungal populations being thrown out of balance.   If this is the case, and if the disrupter is a bacterium, an antibacterial drug may help to restore order.   Sometimes, however, an antibacterial may kill off populations of beneficial bacteria, making matters worse.   Occasionally, as with tetracycline in horses, an antibacterial drug may itself be the disrupter and cause serious disease.

What comes out of all this is that the traditional bad guy germ theory of disease causation is inadequate.   It is not wrong.   It has been helpful in explaining and treating many diseases.   But it is becoming apparent that in treating disease and, especially, in preventing it, going after the bad guy just isn't enough.   In fact, this cowboy approach to medicine tends to lead us into a full-scale war on nature herself -- and there is little doubt as to who will win.

As early as 2400 years ago, Hippocrates wrote:

"Whoever wishes to investigate medicine properly should proceed thus: in the first place consider the seasons of the year, and what effects each of them produces.   Then the winds, the hot and the cold, especially such as are common to all countries, and then such as are peculiar to each locality.   In the same manner, when one comes into a city to which he is a stranger, he should consider its situation, how it lies as to the winds and the rising of the sun; for its influence is not the same whether it lies to the north or the south, to the rising or to the setting sun.   One should consider most attentively the waters which the inhabitants use, whether they be marshy or soft, or hard and running from elevated and rocky situations, and then if saltish and unfit for cooking; and the ground, whether it be naked and deficient in water, or wooded and well watered, and whether it lies in a hollow, confined situation, or is elevated and cold; and the mode in which inhabitants live, and what are their pursuits, whether they are fond of drinking and eating to excess, and given to indolence, or are fond of exercise and labour."

It does not take much imagination to apply Hippocrates' admonitions to the study of animal diseases.   The kinds of factors he refers to are now called "contributing" or "predisposing" causes of disease.   They tend to complicate the neat cause-effect diagrams in which some modern medical scientists want to believe.   Only now, with the aid of modern statistical methods and computers, are these multifarious webs of disease causation being subjected to any kind of scientific scrutiny.   Their undeniable presence means that we can't sit back with our thumbs tucked behind the two holsters of antibiotics and vaccinations.   We need to pay attention to the quality of the air and the water, the nature of the food, and the adequacy of housing.   In agriculture, this is a lesson that needs to be learned again and again.   This is not, as I have heard some suggest, "going backwards" or being "unsophisticated".   If anything, incorporating notions of ecological harmony into our simplistic notions of disease is considerably more sophisticated than the old one-ill one-pill theories.   If there is one thing nature is clear about, it is that if we do not care for her, in the full, patient, loving sense of that word, then she will not cure for us, neither our particular diseases, nor the more general distemper which plagues our times.

EGGSASPERATION: THE OLD SOFT SHELL PROBLEM

A chicken farmer whose hens lay soft-shelled or shell-less eggs is a chicken farmer in trouble. Handling an egg without a shell is not much different, nor more desirable, than handling rooster sperm. Try it some time. Except for not being square, an egg with a shell is a paragon of efficient packaging, an ideal to emulate by "green" businesspeople. On the other hand, the non-square shape of the egg gives it a sensual quality suitable for both children's viewing at Easter and as a focus for mature meditation on life, death, and the esthetics of nature. It is worth a few moments to consider this wonder of nature.

Columbus, when confronted with the challenge of standing an egg on its end, is said simply to have crushed the oval into an upright position on the table. Cheating, some would say, but it worked.

For those who would produce their own eggs, Columbus is not the most exemplary role model: among the possible solutions to laying problems, there are no shortcut cures. Hens tend to lay unusual eggs both very early and very late in life, but correcting the problem of soft shells from a flock of layers in their prime may require an understanding of the process by which an egg is formed and the factors which affect the final result.

By the 17th day of embryonic life, a female chick has more primary oocytes (potential eggs) in her ovary than she will ever again possess. From a peak of 700,000 or so, she drops to around half a million at birth. It's downhill all the way.

When the pullet reaches sexual maturity at around 22 weeks (this varies for different kinds of chickens), one egg develops per day. Each egg requires about 11 days to mature from a pinpoint to full ovulation size. In practice, this means that if birds are knocked out of production it may take 11 days to bring them back into normal laying patterns.

Ovulation is induced by a luteinizing hormone, which itself can be influenced by a number of factors including light. Laying birds should therefore not be subjected to decreasing daylight at the start of their productive life. This can be a problem for birds that start laying in the fall; they will generally do poorly unless provided with artificial light to extend their day to 14 hours or so.   Commercial egg producers will sometimes start their birds on 11 hours of light at 20 weeks and increase the light by 15 minutes a week to as high as 18 hours.   The brightness of the light is not crucial, but the quality is important.   For purposes of sexual stimulation (in chickens, anyway), orange and red lights are said to be most effective.

Light of a different sort is important for another reason. Ultraviolet light, provided by sunlight or fluorescent lights, stimulates the production of vitamin D in the bird's body.   If birds are not subjected to natural or fluorescent light, they will need a vitamin supplement or they will most definitely run into problems with soft shells.   Vitamin D3 is essential for calcium utilization.

The ovary of an actively laying hen is a cluster of follicles (yolks) at varying stages of development.   On the eleventh day of development, the follicle manifests a bloodless line called a stigma, which indicates the site of rupture.   If for some reason a "mistake" is made and the rupture extends beyond the stigma, one of the tiny blood vessels on the follicle may tear, resulting in a bloodspot. Bloodspots are not considered fit for human consumption by the Quality Experts, but for aesthetic reasons only.   The colour of the yolk itself is affected by natural pigments (carotenoids) in the hen's diet.   Saskatchewan birds fed wheat have lighter yolks than Ontario birds fed corn, for instance, but this does not reflect any regional disparity in the nutritional value of eggs.   Egg producers in some parts of the world have suggested adding artificial dye to the chickens' diet in order to cater to social prejudices about yolk colours, having decided that this may be less costly than public education.

Free of the ovary, the yolk drops into a mouth bounded by puckered lily-like lips of tissue called the infundibulum.   Yolks which miss the mouth are usually resorbed and hens which do this consistently are termed internal layers.   (Farmers have called them other names, but it remains to be demonstrated that internal laying is a conscious effort on the part of the hen to thwart her captors.) Once swallowed through the neck of the infundibulum, the yolk is coated with thick albumen (the white) in the portion of the oviduct called the magnum.   Secretion of the white may be stimulated by any irritation in the magnum and, occasionally, tiny eggs with some foreign particle replacing the yolk are laid.   In relatively short order, the egg then receives a thin cloak of membranes, is plumped out with watery albumen, and passes into the uterus (shell gland) where it is destined to spend some 20 of its 24 hours in the outward passage.

The quality of eggshells can be affected by some infectious diseases, by shock, genetic inheritance, age of the bird, or by panting in very hot weather, which changes the acidity of the blood and inhibits one of the chemical reactions involved in shell production. Magner's *Standard Horse and Stock Book* (1912) suggests a simple, though unhelpful, cause of soft shells. "If the ovary matures yolks faster than the latter part of the oviduct does shell, there will be soft-skinned eggs."

By far the most common sources of eggshell quality problems are deficiencies in vitamin D and calcium. I've already discussed Vitamin D. Each eggshell requires about two grams of calcium which must be provided in the laying hens' diet. Cracked oyster shell and limestone chips are commonly used sources of dietary calcium. A fine grind does not alter calcium content, but the birds may not eat it. The pieces should be large enough so that the birds can peck them up, rather than having to stoop to scoop. A coarser grind will be held in the gizzard (muscular stomach) where it has a timed-release effect.

Phosphorus is important for the internal regulation of calcium in the hen, from stomach to bones to eggshells, but most grain-based diets contain adequate phosphorus and this element is not commonly a culprit in shell quality problems. In the end, unless you are willing to spend money on having the chickens' ration analyzed, you may still be stuck with adding a vitamin and/or mineral mix to plug the holes in a problem diet -- or find a special market niche for soft-shelled eggs: "Eggs that are kind to the hen's cloaca". As with most things in nature, it's only bad because we make it so.

SKINNY LEGS, HOT GENES

Moral admonitions to children not to become infatuated with their cousins invariably fall back on tales of the mentally retarded offspring which will undoubtedly arise from even an imagined union of such closely related beings. Nature being all of a piece, and children being naturally inquisitive, one might well be led to ponder the genetic fate of a backyard chicken flock that is limited to the services of only one rooster. Well, some of us, whose minds continue to wander in the afterlight of a prolonged childhood, might be led to ponder such a thing. Does the flock eventually become retarded or susceptible to disease as its inbred line deteriorates? Or are chickens too stupid to lose any more I.Q. points?

Loss of intelligence is rarely a matter of much urgency for the chicken breeder. Imagine, if you will, the lowly hen, head cocked, scratching in the dust. Imagine, then, her set upon, impaled with much indignant squawking and flying of feathers, by a sprinting rooster. There is no doubt what business it is we are concerned with: compulsory copulation, the prolific laying of eggs, and the accretion of succulent flesh. How much flesh and how many eggs, and what comes out of those eggs, are the concerns of poultry geneticists. Even the copulation has, in many cases, been usurped by artificial insemination technicians.

The genetic potential and limitations of the domestic chicken have, over the past two decades, been increasingly controlled and defined by fewer than a dozen multinational corporations -- corporations with names like Shaver, Cobb, De Kalb and Babcock. These companies control most of the layer and broiler production in the Western world. Through rigorous genetic selection, corporate scientists have developed strains of superbird that provide top performance under the high density, atmosphere controlled, mass-production methods used by modern poultry producers. The basic genetic materials -- the grandparent strains of bird -- are among the most closely guarded treasures anywhere on earth. The birds that are released to multipliers or distributors (often part of the same vertically integrated system as the parent breeding companies) are already crossbred and hence not true breeding.

We do know a few things about these chickens. They are quite far removed, for instance, from the wild and vigorous Javanese fowl that are said to be the ultimate source for all our domestic chickens. Most common egg-laying birds are strains of White Leghorn; broiler birds claim Cornish-type fathers and White Plymouth Rock-type mothers. The layers are bred to perform well for one season using limited office space and eating institutional food. The broiler birds are bred to grow fast, be conscripted and sent to slaughter at seven to nine weeks.

All of this would be irrelevant to the backyard poultry fancier if it were not that the birds most readily available to him or her are derived from these very specialized genetic stocks. A bird that thrives in downtown Toronto may not like the food or living quarters in backyard Beaverlodge. They certainly are totally unfit to compete with the scavenging village chickens of Indonesia, who can live on nothing and still, sometimes anyway, outrun a diesel truck. Birds that are bred to reach optimum fatness at seven weeks may just decide to retire at three months if given a stay of the death sentence. Inbreeding uncovers or "concentrates" genes (it does not create new ones) and, as such, it may bring out the worst as well as the best in an animal. Inbreeding can result in a deterioration of reproductive fitness, egg and sperm output, maternal ability, growth rate and hardiness. Using birds of an already refined genetic make-up, this process may be accelerated. If one pushed one's luck, one might even stumble over a strain of epileptic birds such as can be found at the University of Saskatchewan. They are medically both interesting and useful, but somewhat kinky as homestead barnfellows.

In order to avoid the pitfalls of inbreeding, it would be wise to use unrelated sires (roosters) each generation. Those with a conscience sensitized to the evils of corporate control would do well to search out those poultry fanciers who maintain small flocks of what I've heard called "exotics," but which are really just birds that have fallen by the wayside during the development of the Big White Corporate Bird. These outsiders include Barred Plymouth Rocks, Wyandottes, Rhode Island Reds, Hungarian Reds and New Hampshires, and can be found by visiting poultry displays at agricultural fairs or by checking the classified ads in rural weekly newspapers. By keeping this varied genetic stock alive, homesteaders may be doing all of our children a favour; who can predict which genes will be needed for survival by future chickens in the post cheap energy world?

The serious homestead chicken breeder may want to consider developing two separate inbred lines, each of which is superior in different traits. It is important in this case to aim only for those traits considered important; the more targets aimed for, the less likely any one of them is going to get hit. The two inbred lines, once established, may then be crossed to produce birds which, it is hoped, would be superior to both parents.   This increased hardiness and all-round better performance in crossbreds is called hybrid vigour by geneticists and adolescent cockiness by parents.

The societal caution not to wed one's siblings does indeed have relevance even to chickens.   Close, incestuous matings should be avoided when developing inbred lines.   This has nothing do with religion, but relates to what I said earlier about uncovering bad as well as good traits.   The faster this process is carried out, the more likely one is to run into problems.

"Culling", the farmers' euphemism for the last being first into the stewpot for your feast, is one of the most difficult aspects of upgrading a flock, especially the free-running barnyard variety.   Which ones are laying the most eggs?   Growing the fastest? Aristotle, the Greek philosopher, had some opinions on the subject which he expressed in a book titled *The Generation of Animals*.   Prolific egg layers, he said, are "bulky in build, their stomach is hot and very good at concoction, and, in addition, they can easily get at their food . . . the thinness and weakness of their legs contribute towards making these birds prone to copulation and prolific -- and this also applies to human beings.   The nourishment which was intended for the legs is in such cases diverted to the seminal residue." The personality of the bird was also related to its fecundity, according to Aristotle.   A cuckoo didn't lay many eggs because "it is cold by nature (as its cowardice clearly shows)."

While Aristotle's ideas on the subject are interesting, since they are at the foundations of much modern philosophical thought, the last couple of thousand years of experience have produced more reliable criteria for farmers to judge whether or not a chicken is a good layer.   Comb and wattles will be large, smooth, full and waxy in the producing bird.   Her feathering will be trim, her vent large, moist and slightly pink, her pubic bones flexible and at least three fingers apart, and her abdomen soft and pliable.   High producing hens also tend to be late and rapid moulters.

The bottom line in all of this must surely be how much time and attention the homesteader is willing to devote to his or her gallinaceous friends.   One might bed led to ask the question as to how a single-minded devotion to the betterment of chickens reflects on the state of mind of the devotee.   For most small-flock farmers, a minimum of attention to management and culling, and the periodic influx of hot, vigorous new rooster semen will be all that is needed to produce a genetically healthy flock.

SUDDEN DEATH IN DUCKS

A few years ago, a farmer in southern Ontario was watching his two Cayuga and four Pekin ducks swimming in the icy creek flowing through his property. Suddenly one of them, a large young Pekin female, tipped over on to her side and floated downstream. Stopped by some ice, she struggled for several minutes before her head fell down to the cold white surface. The farmer brought her ashore where, despite a chest massage, the duck died. Why, the farmer asked me, did she die? Was it a heart attack? Was it the shock of the cold water? You must understand that a farmer's "why" is not necessarily the same as that of a parent or friend when a loved one dies. Of course, there is that element of caring for the animal in and of itself. But there is more: if we know "why" for this one, perhaps we can prevent another. It is an outward-looking, community-based "why", not an inward-looking, self-absorbed "why". In human community terms, we would say that this is not a "why" based on individual rights, but a "why" based on social justice.

Having said all that, the truth is that we shall never know why the farmer's duck died. Nevertheless, in sound medical and veterinary tradition, I shall not allow such a trivial fact to hinder my imaginings on why she might have died. Medical training allows one to say "I don't know" by such a circuitous route that the client/patient cannot fail to be impressed by it.

The duck could have died from something like a heart attack, but the cold water probably had nothing to do with it. Ducks are much too well protected to be bothered by that sort of thing.

Poisons -- rodenticides, insecticides and the like -- could kill a duck, but I shall assume that it was nothing so obvious.

Many infections can either cause sudden death, or give the illusion of causing sudden death if the animals are not watched too closely. Some individuals just seem to put up with whatever is eating at them until they drop dead. In this case, if it were duck plague or viral hepatitis or some other devastating infection, I would wonder why only one of the six birds was struck down.

Botulism is more accurately, an intoxication than an infection, and early spring is the "wrong" season for it (if disease can be said, in the spirit of Ecclesiastes, to have a right season), but it deserves some discussion if only because it can be an important devastator of waterfowl.   In 1952, some 4 million birds were estimated to have succumbed to botulism in western North America.   Botulism toxin (the same as that which produces paralysis in people) is produced by microorganisms of the same family that produce tetanus (many species), blackleg (cattle, sheep), red water (cattle), black disease (sheep), pulpy kidney disease and lamb dysentery (sheep) and *Clostridium perfringens* food poisoning and gas gangrene in people.   They are a nasty bunch indeed.

What you need for the start of a good botulism outbreak is something dead.   Just about anything will do: insects, fish, birds, rodents.   The spores of the clostridial organisms live in the soil.   They are, with variations due to soil, climate and so on, ubiquitous.   In warm, decaying matter, the spores germinate.   The organisms reproduce, and botulism toxin is produced.   For argument's sake, we'll say that one duck eats a dead insect infected with botulism.   Within 12 hours or so, the duck loses the power of her wings, her legs and finally her neck (limberneck is a common nickname for the disease).   Thereafter the duck departs from her body for that final great migration.   Maggots, those nasty fly babies and no respecters of mortuarial niceties, grow in the body, concentrate the toxin, and are fed on by the other ducks.   Two to three intoxicated maggots can kill a duck.   Presto: death is having his day.   Since these sorts of outbreaks are often associated with shallow, unstable waterlines in late summer, the disease is best prevented by changing the contours of lakes and ponds so that they have sharply dropping shorelines, by minimizing changes in water level and/or keeping the water flowing.   Needless to say, the animal's body should be disposed of.

Other factors related to the diet may do a mortal in.   Acute dietary deficiencies of certain vitamins or minerals could conceivably strike down the fastest growing members of the flock.   These could logically show up at the end of the winter when ducks have been without their bug supplements for several months.   Also a danger at the end of a cool, wet winter are the moulds that grow on grain.   One in particular, the common mould *Aspergillus flavus,* rates dishonourable mention.

In the early 1960s, in England, 100,000 turkey poults died suddenly from a mysterious disease labelled, in a fit of wild imagination, *turkey x* disease.   The perpetrator of this mass kill was found hiding in the feed, a toxin produced by some mould growing on a batch of imported peanut meal.   The mould was *A. flavus,* the toxin, aflatoxin.   It was later discovered that ducks are even more sensitive than turkeys to the effects of aflatoxins.   What is certainly worse, however, is that probably no species is immune to the toxins' deadly effects.   Aflatoxins are said to be the most potent carcinogens, on a per weight basis, known to man (though I confess that I've heard that "scientific" judgement once too often to trust it entirely).   They also cause deformities in the fetus, liver disease, hemorrhages and slow growth.   The toxins are odourless, colourless and not destroyed by ordinary processing such as cooking.   *A. flavus* grows best on cottonseed, corn, peanuts and sorghum.   It might be in your peanut butter; it might be in the corn your ducks are eating.   Aflatoxicosis is a disease of international trade and long-term storage -- a disease of civilization.   There is no cure.   If ever there were an argument for using locally grown produce and paying heed to proper storage, this is it.   No one, I might add, has yet convinced me that the risks of eating peanut butter outweigh the pleasures (ah, the weakness of the flesh).   'Tis better to have eaten peanut butter and died than not to have eaten peanut butter at all.

One dead animal is never much to go on, especially if it dies quickly.   A post mortem rarely reveals anything remarkable in sudden death causes.   The large-scale producers live with their "normal," unaccounted for deaths.   Which is to say, you could be feeding clean corn with a vitamin supplement, quickly dispose of dead animals along the pond's edge, never keep any poisons around, and still have the occasional animal die on you.   For me as a veterinarian, and perhaps for all of us, it may just be Nature reminding us what our ultimate limits are.

CREATION AND EXTINCTION: A MEDITATION

I have a confession to make. I am a terrible naturalist. I cannot name the plants and the animals, even in my back yard. When I go for a walk in the woods, I marvel at the profusion of life, the trees and shrubs and beetles and squirrels and birds -- but without my Audubon guide books and my son Matthew, even sometimes with them, I am incapable of naming them. My wife cringes over my confusions with flowers, how when I first met her I would talk about Rhododendrons, when what I really meant was Marigolds. I mean, she knew that. I was just momentarily confused, a poet overcome by beauty.

I am part of a massive collective failure on the part of modern humanity. We, and we alone in this living biosphere, have been given the task of naming, and of mastery. The task may be unasked for and unwanted, but it is our task, the task of evolution become conscious of itself. Recently, a friend suggested to me that one interpretation of the Genesis account of creation was that we are called upon to develop the kind of mastery over nature that a fine craftsperson has over her material, or a chess master over his game. It is a mastery that begins with a deep understanding of the nature, limitations and possibilities, of the material. We have the role in this Gaia, this living, whole being of which we are but one part, of naming and understanding. I like that. It appeals to me. And then I realize the profundity of my failure -- of our failure -- as the children of the Creator Spirit.

What have we done? We have turned our minds away from Emmanual's Ground, and from the tasks we have been given. We have pretended that we do not really have this task, that we are not really part of creation, that we are some special beings, set here for . . . for what? To act like a bunch of thugs, killing what we cannot name. Like purposeless teenagers in the inner city, we have swarmed the mystery, plundering what we have been given to understand. We have buried ourselves in the stupidity of Biblical, economic and political literalisms and liberal evasions. We have pretended that we can have a theology and an ethic that does not take into account the whole of the natural world, that what is natural has no relevance to what is right, that we can with impunity break the bones and disembowel the living body of which we are a part, that the intellectual games of theologians and philosophers of the last few thousand years are all that matters.

Some scientists estimate that we are losing about one species of living thing from this planet every fifteen minutes -- that we will lose more than a million different creatures over the next 25 years.   The more species we lose, the simpler our task; that many fewer things to name, to understand.   But every part of creation has a role here, and if we drive them from this garden, then we ourselves must take on that role.   At the end of the universe, we shall be called upon to sing not only the song of humanity, but the song of the auroch and the quagga, the giant lemur, the Carolina parakeet, the glyptodont, the moa, and perhaps (hopefully not -- is there not enough already?) the elusive snow leopard, the delicately beautiful golden lion tamarin, and the hauntingly massive blue whale.   We shall be called upon to sing the songs of all those creatures whose songs we have silenced before we ever heard them.

As I noted at the beginning of this book, according to some Jewish legends and commentaries (the Midrash), there have been multiple creations, either simultaneous with our own, or preceding it.   In the last few decades, scientists have accumulated much evidence documenting the history of the earth as a history of extinction and resurrection.   In fact, extinction has already claimed some 99% of all species that have ever lived, many of them through periodic mass die-offs.   I wish I could go back in time with you three or four billion years and, like some bishop in a Latin American dictatorship, walk you through the lists of the disappeared, to name them, the crinoids and the ammonoids, the trilobites and the ammonites, names like those of Middle-eastern desert tribes of biblical times, to give the date and the time of their disappearance.

But as I have already said, I'm terrible at remembering names and though as an epidemiologist I spend my life counting things and statistically analyzing populations some numbers are beyond my humble mind.   A billion years, or a few million -- how can I conceive of those things? I have trouble remembering last week, or imagining the limits of my few brief years on earth.   I sometimes wish I had the arrogance of an evolutionist or a creationist, that I understood the mind of the Creator, or the body of Gaia, that I could confuse absolutely and without embarrassment the mechanisms of how with the mysteries of why.   Why does order come from chaos? Why are certain molecular configurations more stable than others?   Why does oxygen react with hydrogen to produce water, and with carbon to make fire?   Why is there a sister death star, or a wobble in the galaxy, or whatever, to periodically bring showers of rocks or comets to earth? Why are there shifts in the earth's tectonic plates, creating new continents and volcanoes and climates? Why, not how, at some molecular or sub-molecular level, as if atomic particles must be inherently so. I am not satisfied with subatomic descriptions of how or religious *ex cathedra* statements of why. I want to know why, really?

Why is the slate sometimes wiped almost clean? Our arrogance, maybe?

Archaeologists are now telling us that every major wave of death in Gaia -- these mass extinctions that come every 25-35 million years -- is followed by a tremendous profusion of new life forms, that the rules of evolution are suddenly changed, that what was previously advantageous is no longer of any use: gills out of water, heat-loss mechanisms in an ice-age, fur in the tropics. In the face of water loss from the atmosphere in beginning times, photosynthesis using water was born, in the crucible of toxic oxygen, the symbiosis of respiring bacteria, from the graveyard of the dinosaurs, the flowering of primates.

Gaia, the embryonic life of which we are a part, grows on, adapts, changes -- just as we grow and change even as thousands of our body cells die and are replaced. Am I the child that once was? Well, yes and no. Who were the 12-year-old Hildi Froese and David Toews who met at the Bronx Park skating rink in Winnipeg one evening in 1960 or the Dorothy Friesen with whom I pushed my baby sister Irene around in 1955? People I once knew, still in here, in there somewhere, I suppose. Is this creation around us the primal creation? Well, no of course not. Where are the original bacteria, the green scums of a billion years ago and the monsters of a mere million? Well, yes, of course, the constituents of every living thing are still here; the bacteria live on in us, in the growling fermentations of our pre-prandial guts, and the dancing of the neural impulses across our *corpus callosa.*

But if extinctions occur -- and resurrections -- every few tens of millions of years, and if the body of creation lives on, what business is it of ours to meddle with the current wave of extinctions? What is different now?

Rick Gore, one of the assistant editors of *National Geographic* magazine, writes in the June 1989 issue of his dismay at climbing up the "overgrazed scrubland" on the slopes of a Hawaiian volcano. Is this barren landscape of pigs, cactuses and rats a vision of our global future? he asks.   Delving into his anger at this wasted land, he asks what makes our current devastation different from those that have come before.

"We are the difference," he concludes.   "For the first time since life on earth began four billion years ago, a living organism can begin to understand what is happening to this planet.   We can see that the health of species is interconnected, that if we let too many disappear, we will go too.   For the first time, a living organism can consciously do something to halt a mass extinction.   Perhaps most important, for the first time a living creature can gaze out across the species of the earth and say: This is beautiful.   I care.   I will not let it go."

Modern humanity's dejectedness at the desolation we are causing is an echo of words spoken by the Jewish prophet Jeremiah, who describes a terrible desolation, a kind of de-creation:

I saw the earth, and it was without form and void:
the heavens, and their light was gone.
. . .
I saw, and the farm-land was wilderness,
and the towns all razed to the ground.
. . .
These are the words of the Lord:
The whole land shall be desolate,
though I will not make an end of it.

The whole land desolate -- but not completely: it almost seems as if the apocalyptic-prophetic tradition is a re-statement, in various historical contexts, of the ancient history of the earth -- and of our future?

More to the point of our discussion here, however, are the following words, which he adds to his tales of judgement and desolation: "But your wrongdoing has upset nature's order, and your sins have kept you from her kindly gifts." We are used to thinking about sin as an individual act -- murder, gluttony, theft, betrayal -- and punishment, as well, as individual. Salvation and hell are personal. And yet suffering of individuals in this life bears no relationship to their virtue. We know this. We don't really need a prophet or God to remind us, do we?

And yet we live with this ambiguity: that, although personal fate is not tied to personal virtue, we, collectively, will suffer for our wrongdoings.   Collective murder, gluttony, theft, betrayal -- these are the sins of humanity against creation.   And yes, the sins of the parents are visited on the children, and as we sow, *as a people*, so indeed shall we reap. While it is not fashionable to say that Marxism was right in some things, I think few would dispute the Marxist insight that many of the evils (poverty, environmental degradation) once ascribed to otherwordly forces (acts of God or Satan) are more likely the natural consequences of the cynical deeds of people.

If we think in geological time, which is a bit like theological time (a million years in a day, and a day in a million years) can we safely say that we are in our last day? Are we like a barren fig tree inviting the Gardener to cut us down, like a cancerous growth in Gaia, bringing down upon ourselves the inevitable immunological rejection, the one we have seen in wave upon wave of creation, the uprooting of ourselves, the global immune system engulfing us and cleaning us out?

St. Paul speaks of the whole created universe groaning in expectation of a new heaven and a new earth. As he saw it, the new heaven and the new earth shall come out of this one, not be created *ex nihilo*. If so, perhaps we are looking forward -- after the harvest and the garden cleaning -- to a whole new flowering of creation. Perhaps we shall be there. I believe that, as all previous creations live on in us, we shall live on in the new worlds. But shall we be there as people, as redeemed, distinct, entities? Unless we change our ways, perhaps not.

But change what? All of human life is intricately bound up with the fate of this planet, but in two main ways our relationship reaches the most delicate of intimacies. When we eat, we are taking pieces of the world around us and putting them into intimate contact with our bodies. Every act of eating can be seen as an act of love -- or of something more brutal, a kind of copulation. This is what makes eating together in courtship, and in families, the Passover meal and the Eucharist such a powerful act of sharing. The sharing is not only symbolic, not only spiritual; from a global creation viewpoint, eating is a real act of trust, vulnerability and sharing. And this is tied up with another intimate act: that of making waste; because what we put out into the environment will come back to us, eventually, in our food. Do we trust our neighbours not to pollute our food? The sustainable production of a safe food supply and the appropriate handling of our dirt seem mundane, prosaic. They are. They are as dull as foot-washing and the breaking of bread. They are what binds us together in trust to each other, to Gaia, and to the Spirit who created us.   The rules of this game which we are called upon to master are, in some ways very simple, and, ultimately, benevolent.

It is therefore precisely in these things -- in how we eat and how we handle our dirt, or waste and sewage -- that we express our faith in a planetary context.   If we hew down the complex forests and fill in marshlands to grow hamburgers and monocultures of wheat or rice or sugar, what does that say? According to the Judeo-Christian myth of creation God gave us -- no, not just us, but all the wild creatures of earth *all* the seed-bearing plants and trees for food (there's no mention of giving us animals for food in the Genesis account, but that's another story).   What does it say when we clean off 99% of the plate and say, "Here, we'll grow these few, for us, with the help of some good poisons to get rid of those other annoying things You've created -- that's good enough.   And I guess the wild animals will have to get by with something less than You'd planned for them." What does this say about us? About how well we're fulfilling our role here? We're fond of the "being fruitful and increasing" part and yes, we've done pretty well at that, but we are called upon for more than simple copulatory multiplication.   Isn't it about time we paid attention to a few of the other things?

I don't want to go off on a tangent about a decentralized, diversified food system, natural foods and the like.   I only want to point out that one doesn't celebrate the beautiful singing of the sopranos by getting rid of the altos.   The beauty is in the relation-ships, the harmonies.   We celebrate creation by celebrating -- in our eating and in our waste management, for lack of a better word -- the complex, diverse harmony of Gaia, the created Living Being.

There's a tendency among some peace activists and environ-mentalists to suffer from a Jonah syndrome.   You know, we cry doomsday scenarios about nuclear war, and suddenly we have a flowering of peace negotiations around the world and our enemies say, "See, the nuclear threat worked" or "The nuclear threat was not as dangerous as we thought.   Everything's going to be all right."   A similar kind of environmental awakening seems to be taking place around the world, as imperfect and slow as the peace awakening, but positive nonetheless.   There are real dangers that we set aside our vigilance, or believe the enemy.   "See, God didn't punish us after all.   The sins didn't matter."   We need to be care-ful not to confuse repentance and forgiveness with what might have happened had we done nothing.   The doomsday prophecies do matter. And we need, urgently it seems to me, to go beyond them. Positive changes in behaviour are to be celebrated. Let's throw a big party for the prodigal wastemongers when they come home -- when Dow Chemical recycles plastic and the city fathers support composting and Ronald Reagan shakes hands with Gorbachov. What better occasion for a party?

When I see positive actions around the world, I think, who knows, maybe there's still hope for me. If 10-year-old Rebecca labelled the rows in the garden right, I can learn about the peas and the beans and the lettuces -- and maybe even the Rhodo*den*drons and that precious, expensive climbing ivy -- what was its name again? I all but eliminated in my eagerness to get out all the weeds from the garden plot. And if 12-year-old Matthew is patient with me, I can learn the names of the bugs in the back yard. It's a long task, one that I should be doing with, literally, religious care. Maybe -- though I read nothing of this in the Bible, and evolutionary biologists will tell me it's heresy -- maybe the virtues of the children can be visited upon the parents?

DAVID WALTNER --TOEWS, DVM

David Waltner-Toews (nee Toews) was born and raised in Winnipeg. He left after one year of university for a stint of hitch-hiking in Europe and overland to Asia, working as a Mennonite Central Committee volunteer in rural India; this was followed by an exploration of Malaysia, Thailand, Laos and Cambodia (now Kampuchea) by bus, foot, train, rice barge and bicycle. On return-ing to Canada, he worked as a sawmill worker in Vancouver and returned to college to complete a degree in English literature (Goshen College). He then hyphenated his name (by marriage) and switched careers.

He earned his DVM from the Western College of Veterinary Medicine in 1978, spent two years in private veterinary practice (in northern Alberta and southern Ontario), and then entered a PhD program in epidemiology at the University of Guelph. During the next five years, besides conducting extensive research work on the management and diseases of dairy calves, Dr. Waltner-Towes worked with other veterinarians on disarmament, disaster medicine, inter-national development, and environmental issues, particularly in agriculture.

Between 1985-87, he worked as an epidemiologist on a project to build an animal disease investigation centre for the islands of Java and Madura in Indonesia. He returned as a faculty member to the University of Guelph in 1987, where he teaches courses in the epidemiology of zoonoses and the epidemiology of food-borne diseases, and on "The Global Ecology of Veterinary Medicine". He is involved in epidemiologic research projects on animal produc-tion and health, zoonotic diseases, and environmental issues.

He has been actively involved in international programs, in-cluding a Graduate Diploma in International Veterinary Medical Development, and institutional strengthening programs with the veterinary schools in Costa Rica and Columbia. He has been the project coordinator to provide technical support to 14 Caribbean countries to develop a computerized animal and plant health infor-mation network.

David's publications include scientific papers, four books of poetry, and numerous short stories and essays. He is, by his own admission, interested in everything on the planet, and regrets only that he has but lifetime (that he remembers anyway) to take it all in.